Emma Markezic has been a writer, j[...] comedian for well over a decade. Milli[...] on topics as far-reaching as sex, feminism, fitness, fashion, wellness and current affairs.

She's written for global titles including *Vogue*, *Marie Claire*, *Good Housekeeping*, *Sunday Telegraph*, *InStyle*, *GQ*, *Woman's Day*, *Who*, *Elle*, Buzzfeed and more.

She's performed in the Melbourne International Comedy Festival, told jokes on *Studio 10*, was awarded Rising Star in *Cosmopolitan*'s Women of the Year Awards in 2010, and once said 'Did you eat a sexy beast this morning?' on *60 Minutes*.

In 2016 she was diagnosed with aggressive breast cancer. She lost her hair but not her head, something which eventually led to the birth of this book.

She lives in ... well, who cares really. She lives.

HarperCollins*Publishers*

Curveballs.

**how to keep it together
when life tries to tear
you a new one.**

Emma
Markezic

HarperCollins*Publishers*

First published in Australia in 2019
by HarperCollins*Publishers* Australia Pty Limited
ABN 36 009 913 517
harpercollins.com.au

HarperCollins*Publishers*

Level 13, 201 Elizabeth Street, Sydney NSW 2000, Australia
Unit D1, 63 Apollo Drive, Rosedale, Auckland 0632, New Zealand
A 53, Sector 57, Noida, UP, India
1 London Bridge Street, London, SE1 9GF, United Kingdom
Bay Adelaide Centre, East Tower, 22 Adelaide Street West, 41st floor, Toronto,
  Ontario M5H 4E3, Canada
195 Broadway, New York NY 10007, USA

A catalogue record for this book is available from the National Library of Australia

ISBN 978 1 4607 5526 6 (paperback)
ISBN 978 1 4607 0960 3 (ebook)

Cover design by Darren Holt, HarperCollins Design Studio
All illustrations by the author
Typeset in Sabon LT Std by Kirby Jones
Printed and bound in Australia by McPherson's Printing Group
The papers used by HarperCollins in the manufacture of this book are a natural,
recyclable product made from wood grown in sustainable plantation forests. The fibre
source and manufacturing processes meet recognised international environmental
standards, and carry certification.

To you, for buying this book.
But also Big Z, for being a dude.

CONTENTS

This just in: World not oyster after all

What happens when you step on one of the great Lego pieces of life? When you get blind-sided. Sucker-punched. Or just stuck in a big, fat rut. Because you will, eventually. You'll get divorced. Or fired. Or cancer. And, just quietly ... that's not what we were promised.

Many of us were told we could be whatever we wanted. Do whatever we wanted. Do *whoever* we wanted while having whatever nose we wanted. For the first time in human history, we had it all. Chicken nuggets had arrived, *Doogie Howser* was on TV and life was good.

Yet, despite this utopia, we still need motivational quotes just to get through the day. And I happen to have a pretty colossal problem with motivational quotes. Namely if it fits inside an Instagram square, I'm rather dubious about its ability to change your life. Or even your afternoon.

But we're liking and we're sharing, which means we're searching for something – something, I suspect, far more than

1

the diarrhoea-like procession of cyber encouragement we get via social media. Something to help us cope with a life those euphoric childhoods of twilight bike rides and Easter egg hunts left us woefully unprepared for. In short, we're searching for the ability to deal with a big, fat let-down. When our business fails. When we're not married by thirty. When we get sick. When someone dies. When life suddenly isn't the Happy Meal-having, saccharine-sweet ride we were promised. Because at some point, it won't be. Trauma happens every day, to everyone. The only difference between you and the next guy is how you deal with the curveballs that come your way.

This was the conclusion I came to when it happened to me. When I was diagnosed with cancer and had to learn to like it or lump it. Quite literally. What I found, to my surprise, was that I had an innate ability to manage the onslaught better than some people seem to manage a paper cut. I wondered if I was perhaps just mentally stronger – the way some people are more physically gifted, like born athletes or natural ballerinas? I'm certainly neither of those things, but curveball wrangling turns out to be something I can do with aplomb. And since it seems rather selfish to keep this decidedly mad skill to myself, I wanted to find a way to share how I did it. How I survived. How anyone can be Teflon to trauma, if they have the right tools.

So I spent the last twelve months researching it – speaking to experts, listening to stories. Investigating why some people seem to be more psychologically resilient than others and figuring out how we can all train ourselves to be more unfuckwithable, cancer or no cancer. I've taken all the best bits and condensed them down to eighteen techniques you can do today, tomorrow and every day for the rest of your life. A veritable stock cube for living anxiety-free, if you will. A recipe that you can refer back to again and again, supported by science and designed to help you handle your own curveballs with grace, humour and pluck.

Each of the actions I've laid out are things I did to get myself through the worst time in my life. Maybe they won't all work for you – pick and choose the ones that do, and discard the rest. There's no right or wrong way out of agony. It's an incredibly personal ride. It's true that what doesn't kill you makes you more interesting at parties – but in the meantime, try these. Because they're the easiest, most effective, most soul-affirming ways to get through this life that I know.

Because it turns out you *can* learn to keep it together when life tries to tear you a new one. And what's more, you can have a lot of fun while doing it.

But first ... a story.

NEED-TO-KNOWS

Everything you need to know about
happiness, pain, grief, curveballs and
a guy named Fats Bam Bam.

CHAPTER ONE

Finding Freda
(Or: Why I'm qualified to talk about curveballs)

It's fair to say a woman's rack looks sublime in a push-up bra. Like a Jeff Koons balloon sculpture rendered in flesh. A verse of physical poetry. This story begins with boobs, is what I'm saying.

Mine, funnily enough. They were gathered together in one such bra I'd purchased just the day before. I was at a wedding in Asheville, North Carolina. A very Southern wedding, if the moonshine and hay bales were anything to go by. All the people saying 'y'all' without a crumb of irony was entrancing for a girl from Australia who'd never even heard of 'shrimp and grits' before, let alone eaten them for three days straight with a peach cobbler chaser. The bride had shed her heels, the groom had loosened his tie and there was a ten-piece big band playing across the room. There were drums and tubas and a guy hitting a mason jar with a stick. The saxophone player in particular had piqued my interest and I was fixin' to make a move.

As it happens, I'd been dating a guy at home in Australia for a few months but it was one of those nonsensical non-exclusive arrangements you hear so much about. A millennial special, if you will. For my part, I'd never so much as looked at two men at the same time before, so this felt like the ideal time to give it a whirl. There was just something about the curve of the sax player's instrument which really buttered my corn.

I pondered which Southern-themed pick-up line would sound best in an Australian accent. 'You look like you've been ridden hard and put away wet' was the one I landed on. He was awfully sweaty after all and it felt right, if a little cheesy. Before making my way over to deliver this linguistic artistry, I attempted to readjust the body parts I'd already shoehorned into the Victoria's Secret special I'd purchased for the occasion.

And that's when it happened. It felt like a frozen pea floating in custard. A notion gross enough on its own, but this was far worse. There was a lump in the middle of my left breast.

You already know that little nugget was cancer. Not least of which because I mentioned it in the intro, but also because we rarely use the word 'breast' unless it's medical: breast exam, breast augmentation, breast cancer. In recreational life, we're far more attuned to boobs, titties, fun bags.

Still, I didn't know it at the time. And while the discovery of the lump that would be cancer sent a shiver through me that made the sequins on my dress do a sort of quivering conga line, it was easily dismissed. 'I'm sure it's nothing,' I told myself. 'Maybe it's one of those curious third nipples you always hear about. Or perhaps one of those freaky balled-up twins they sometimes find inside people, made up of teeth and hair.'

Yes, it's a dark day when a parasitic hair twin is at the top of your wish list.

But the brain is an incredibly manipulative thing. And parasitic twin is what I went with that breezy Saturday afternoon in North

Carolina. I danced, I drank, I made out with the saxophone player and I put that lump at the back of my mind for another day.

It's a cavernous place, really – the human mind. You can fit in everything from your top ten favourite *Simpsons* quotes to how to spell *handkerchief* to a precise recollection of the phone number you had when you were eight years old, all without touching the sides. It's little wonder things get lost in there all the time. Not the *Simpsons* quotes, of course, but the other stuff. And the discovery of that lump I pushed deep into the cranial cheap seats where it stayed, somehow completely ignored, for days.

It eventually resurfaced a week later on the flight back to Sydney, where I was living at the time. Right there in seat 23B. Probably because scoring a 'B' seat on an economy flight is the very definition of hell above earth. It meant I was helplessly pinned between a sweaty man-spreader and a woman with a Hello Kitty–emblazoned phone whose small frame belied her gargantuan snore. Since my body couldn't escape, my brain needed to. And so it rifled around for recent additions with a view to distraction.

Ping! There it was. My friend Lumpy McLumpface. I found myself genuinely shocked I'd actually managed to forget about it. A shiver similar to the original overcame me, but with no sequins to make the most of the ensuing ripple, it was a lot less flashy the second time around. Positively chilling, in fact.

A lump. In my breast. That's definitely not great.

Could I have cancer? Of course I could. Anyone could. I'd watched my own father succumb to lung cancer almost two years earlier. And if you've ever watched anyone have their last breath taken from them by the Big C, you know it's not a good time. In fact, I tend to be of the opinion that watching anyone die from a debilitating, degenerative condition is one of the most overwhelming and confusing ordeals in the human repertoire of experience. All at once you're both devastated and relieved. Heartbroken and reconciled. It all came rushing back in an unpleasant avalanche of emotion. Was I going to die from cancer as well? Continue the family tradition?

'Don't be silly,' I could already hear my friends saying. 'You're going to be *fine*.'

But of course, not everyone is fine, are they? People die every day. From all sorts of horrific things. Some of them in far less meaningful ways than others. Like – just for example – a dude named Hans Staininger, who broke his neck when he tripped over his own beard. Or a lawyer named Clement Vallandigham, who shot himself while trying to prove how someone shot himself. And these are just the senseless accidents. What about the fifteen million-odd people globally who will die from a heart attack or stroke this year alone? Things, whether you like it or not, are not always going to be fine.

Still … we don't think it will happen to us, do we?

What made me think I was any different? That I deserved anything more than Hans or Clement or my dad? This wasn't like that throbbing tooth I could probably convince myself to ignore for months on end; this was worth checking out. I'd go see my doctor as soon as I got back, I thought. So he can tell me it's nothing.

With that squared away I still had a good eleven hours of flight time to go, so my brain decided to ruminate on some other things. Like why do bad things always seem to happen in North Carolina, anyway? I'm not superstitious, but as a state I feel it might be cursed. Just look at the evidence:

1. Found lump there.

2. Oral sex is technically still illegal there.

3. Almost every episode of *Dateline* is set there.

It's not an exhaustive list, but still.

After contemplating this for a while, the adrenalin finally started draining away. Eventually I gave into my biology and joined Hello Kitty girl in a nap. I landed on a Saturday night and was at the doctor's office by Monday afternoon to get Freda checked out. Freda was what I had decided to call my parasitic twin, after my first cat.

'Yep, that's a lump all right,' Dr Chang said while groping me with gloved fingers.

Cue third round of full-body shivers.

'Oh, it is? Like ... a for-real lump?'

'Yes. [glove snap] We're going to have to send you off for an ultrasound.'

Deep down I'd expected him to wave me away with a limp hand. 'Geddoutta here, you hypochondriac, you – come back when you're feverish or oozing pus. Shoo now!'

Only he didn't. He wrote me a referral and looked me in the eye a lot.

The ultrasound led to a mammogram, which led to a biopsy. Throughout the whole process I tried my best to keep it light.

'When I hashtagged "free the nipple", this isn't what I had in mind,' I told the mammogram technician, as she sandwiched my chest into a vice.

Each time I tried to take the edge off the situation like this, I was met with the kind of steely glare only people who have been to law or medical school seem to be able to execute. I saw at least half a dozen different versions of the glare that day, which did not help brighten the mood one bit. I couldn't have felt more uncomfortable if I was Harvey Weinstein at a Women's March. And I imagine that would be relatively excruciating.

Two days later I was back in Chang's examination room, my best friend trailing behind me with a notebook, pen and pocket-size packet of tissues. As soon as the doc leaned over and put his hand on my knee, I knew. It was cancer.

There are only two reasons a doctor will put his hand on your knee, after all, and one could end in jail time. I don't know if the lure of an affair with me would warrant being potentially sodomised in the shower by a guy nicknamed Fats Bam Bam, so I knew it was pretty bad news.

(That's the actual nickname of a man currently serving a life sentence in a Colorado correctional facility, by the way – I wrote to a guy there to get some ideas.)

Actually, I suppose I knew about forty-two hours earlier, when I'd gone to buy a pair of silk pyjamas because I usually sleep naked and figured that would be frowned upon once I was hospitalised. Sometimes you just know.

Chang said the word 'okay' a lot in the ensuing minutes – almost with the expectation it would somehow stop me crying if he checked in at the end of every sentence.

'So it looks like it is cancer, okay?'

Followed by: 'The next step is to get you to see the surgeon, okay?'

And finally: 'Now, how are you feeling – are you feeling … okay?'

No part of this story is particularly unique. Women are diagnosed with breast cancer every day. But what happened next is where things really start to get compelling.

Essentially … nothing happened. Allow me to explain.

A lot of people would use the expression 'my world turned upside down' at this point in the story. Only mine didn't. I walked out, looked at my friend, said, 'Bottle of wine, then?' and we proceeded to get drunk in front of the TV in my apartment, watching Whitney Houston video clips on repeat and singing at the top of our lungs. Everyone deals with these things differently, and apparently I was going to deal with it like it was 1999 and everyone was invited.

There wasn't much I could do at this point, was what I figured. It had happened and I had to deal with the outcome, whatever that would prove to be. Could I die? Sure, that's how cancer works. It wants to survive and thrive just like everything else on the planet. I didn't begrudge it that. In fact, all I really thought with any emphatic certainty was, 'I can do this.' That's it. Just, 'I can do this,' and nothing more.

In a way, this was more shocking than the tumour itself. Who did I think I was not to fall apart at the seams at a cancer diagnosis in my early 30s when I was poor, single and living alone? It's what people expected, even wanted. For a while I assumed it was probably just taking its sweet time – the breakdown, that is. That I'd sail through the first few days only to suddenly snap like a Twix a week later, and find myself uncontrollably sobbing in the supermarket while buying toilet paper and milk.

Instead, a week later I was admitted for a radical mastectomy.

Still, no breakdown.

At this point I assumed it was because it was such a breathtaking timeline that it only gave me just enough wiggle room to throw my doomed organ a 'boobvoyage' and little more. There's nothing like a party to take your mind off things like an impending amputation, after all. And a boob-themed shindig with a handful of close friends was where it felt like my energy should go. As I downed a Slippery Nipple and tucked into a rack of lamb, I couldn't help but think ... should I have served duck breast instead? Had I missed the boat on boob-themed foods here? I mean, you really only get one crack at a boobvoyage. Two at best.

Before I knew it the party was over. And still, no breakdown.

But the surgery was my first and, as such, I wasn't completely prepared for the aftermath. When I woke up, my right hand instinctively clutched at my chest. There was nothing; it was gone. Where a round mass used to be there was just a void. Like a deflated balloon. It felt flat and sore. So very, very sore.

Of course it's sore, I scolded myself. You have a four-inch incision in your chest and they just scooped out your insides like a man helping himself to scrambled eggs at a breakfast buffet. That's going to sting a little.

Still, no breakdown.

A day later, when I managed to haul myself out of bed and assess the damage, I admit it was more macabre than I had imagined. The bruising was akin to a grisly pride flag, all purple and red and yellow and green. My nipple hung there, askew. It was an alien landscape in miniature, all valleys and shadows, unfamiliar and breathtaking. The stitches looked so dark against my pale skin, so jagged.

But even at that point I never asked 'Why me?' Not once. It didn't even occur to me. Not even when the post-operation results came in and my surgeon gently unfolded the origami of my treatment plan one crease at a time. The tumour was bigger than they thought. More aggressive too. Chemo would follow, then likely radiation. I would lose my hair. My sense of taste and smell. My life as I knew it.

Still, even then – in what was probably the darkest hour of my discontent – all I could think was 'I can do this.' That was it. There were very few tears, no existential arguments with the universe and no regrets. I guess that's where the real story began.

You may be asking how this is useful to you – the person who is struggling with something so overwhelming it made you pick up this book. It probably seems the complete opposite of useful, in fact. Like giving a fork to someone eating a bowl of soup. And it's not that I haven't experienced trauma of all kinds in my time. Physical, mental, emotional, the kind that makes your chest tight and your soul ache. The type that feels like it's drained all the water from your cells and somehow changed the colour of the sky itself. I've been there, in those depths. More than once. But somewhere along the way I turned into a Slip'N Slide for misery – and going through cancer treatment shone a light on that fact like a paparazzi bulb on a Kardashian. After that, it readily became my life's goal to show other people how to do it too.

So while you might not have cancer (although with one in two of us now getting it, you may well have), you will have some other monolith casting a shadow over your existence. It might be anxiety or a bad breakup or a miscarriage or all of the above. Maybe you just feel like you're in a rut you can't get out of; that prickly feeling you didn't get the life you were promised. And while I'm not a doctor and can't prescribe you ... well, anything, I can give you the tools you need to deal with life's epic clusterfucks from the ground up. Because at some point we all go from 'No one is going to tell me what to do with my life' to 'Can someone please tell me what to do with my life?!' It happens somewhere between sixteen and thirty-six, generally, to the better of us. The decline from undaunted to unsure is so gradual we don't even know it's happening. But when the doubt sets in, it's like a red wine stain on a white silk shirt. So it's your choice: the agony of staying where you are or the agony of growing through it like a plant pushing through the pavement?

I'm going to go right ahead and assume you chose the second one. Because life is going to suck all the balls, that's just the nature of it. Which is exactly why you need to learn to enjoy it even when the chips are down. You need to scoop up those fries from the bottom of the bag and appreciate them, even though they're lukewarm and soggy. Because life doesn't get easier – you just get stronger.

Cancer taught me a lot – not the least of which is that life isn't unfair at all. It's completely fair because it's unfair to everyone in equal measure. Trauma can come for anyone, at any time. Should you live long and fully, you'll find that some days you'll feel so inflated with love you might burst, and others you'll feel yourself collapsing slowly and pitifully like a piece of abandoned fruit. What I want to teach you is not how to get back to a place of happiness, but rather how to find happiness in everything, even when it feels like your existence has been punctured from the inside out. I promise, it's possible.

Essentially this is a lesson in mining clouds for silver linings, because the underside of each and every one has a metallic belly that's not always obvious from the outset. I can help you find it – I have an uncanny ability to rise to the occasion and I want to teach you how to have it too. Right now, your fear of your life coming up short is probably causing your life to come up short. But we can change that. Trust me ... even my blood type is B positive.

So let's begin.

CHAPTER TWO

The handshake

(Or: Why you don't have to ever get over it)

Some people lead charmed lives; others have to fight for everything they get. Most of us are somewhere in the creamy middle. But we all have to deal with an unwelcome upheaval sooner or later. We often think of trauma as being something dramatic – something that happens during car accidents or as a result of war. Something that pertains to all manner of especially heinous things that would make great episodes of *Law & Order: Special Victims Unit*. But for some people, there's nothing more traumatic than a handshake.

It doesn't exist on a scale, you see. There's no ruler psychologists use to measure your trauma against the next guy's. It's completely and utterly subjective.

That might seem like a cold notion – the idea that your trauma is no less important than that of a thirteen-year-old who just experienced their first breakup. Or that your brother's suicide isn't any more harrowing than your neighbour's houseplant dying. But humans tend to deal with trauma in the same way they deal with humour: you can no more stop yourself laughing at a dirty joke you find amusing than you can feeling traumatised by an event, whatever it may be.

I wasn't ribbing you about the handshake either. There was a man – let's call him Rob. And Rob's life was ruined by a handshake. At least that's what he thought. And as far as trauma goes, that's all that matters.

I know this because I spent a sizeable chunk of time talking to a man called Paul Joseph Stevenson. Paul's seen more suffering in his life than most people have seen blades of grass. He's the Sheriff of Shockingham, in fact, patrolling the Forest of Upheaval, guarding against stress and agony. Or rather (and perhaps more accurately), Paul's an expert in psychological trauma, post-traumatic stress disorder (PTSD) and psychological recovery from disaster incidents. He has counselled survivors of Australia's Port Arthur massacre and Thredbo landslide, the Bali bombings and the Indian Ocean tsunami, and families of passengers from Malaysian Airlines Flight 370, to name just a few horrific incidents. He's also written books about international disaster management and, for my pair of pennies, he is the godfather of restoration. Although I'm also hoping that the Sheriff of Shockingham moniker takes off – I was pretty chuffed when I came up with that.

'In order to survive trauma, it's actually not always possible to integrate everything into our lives,' he tells me after I ponder if maybe we've all just become a bit snowflake-esque in the age of Echo Dots and UberEats. Isn't it possible we just all need to mother the fuck up? (Side note: I've decided 'man the fuck up' should be changed to 'mother the fuck up'. I'm neither a man nor a mother but one definitely looks decidedly harder than the other.)

But Paul assures me no, that's not it at all.

Which brings me back to the handshake. When I asked Paul about the worst trauma he'd ever seen I expected a disturbing story about 9/11 or a family annihilator. But no, it was Rob and his frightful fist-pumping.

'He was on stress leave because a handshake went badly and he'd come to me for counselling,' Paul tells me. 'He'd put his hand out to shake another man's hand and the man rejected him. In his culture, that was a very serious situation for him; he felt he wasn't respected. And so he claimed the way the handshake went wrong caused him anxiety and depression. That may sound unreasonable, but when I actually got to talking to him, he had all the signs and symptoms of a person who was going through trauma.'

Now, you're probably thinking what I first thought when I heard that story: worst worker's comp claim EVER. But that's just your comparison talking.

'It's probably the least traumatic event I can think of personally,' agrees Paul. 'But it still had relatively the same kind of impact as something like an armed robbery or fatal car accident would have on someone else.'

And the same logic goes for what perturbs you – whether it's past sexual abuse, seeing that your ex has moved on or learning you have an STI. Maybe it's just having a guy cut you off at the lights and give you the finger. It doesn't matter what it is. I'll let Paul say it again for extra effect: 'Everybody's trauma is as important as everybody else's, regardless of what it is.'

Which is a fair statement. Why should one person's pain stand above anyone else's?

Here's where it starts to get a little more confusing, though, psychologically speaking – there is absolutely no way to tell what you're going to find traumatic the first time out. You could experience a plane crash and be fine, but find someone making fun of your haircut completely distressing. Even when people experience the *exact same* event, they will have utterly divergent reactions.

'You might have ten people in a fast-food outlet that's just been robbed at gunpoint,' says Paul. 'Two or three of them, they shrug it off and go home and forget about it. Two or three of them will then be mildly or moderately affected, and two or three might be hysterical and extremely traumatised by it. And they've all just witnessed the same event simultaneously.'

What's more, the severity of your response doesn't necessarily change even when the trauma seesaw tips in your direction.

'I've seen people who are incredibly traumatised over a small shunt in the back of the car while they're stationary without any injuries at all; then there are other people who have no trauma having walked away after a multiple rollover. It's really the perception people have of their trauma that counts.'

So where does this individual set point come from? Maybe you're born with it, maybe you dropped a gene?

'The theoretical approach I take says it's based on early amygdala-based trauma, which is the only developed part of the brain in children up to around age four,' says Paul. 'Children, who have a pre-hippocampal brain, will automatically suffer amygdala-based trauma should something happen to them and that's going to stimulate fright, flight or fight.'

So a quick refresh on that high-school anatomy class you no doubt forgot years ago to make way for important things like the lyrics to 'Bohemian Rhapsody': the amygdala is the area of the brain that automatically processes your emotions before you're even really aware of them. Once we become adults, we then go on to consciously react to those feelings. Children, however, don't have that luxury. It's just raw, unfiltered emotion. That's why toddlers are such little boneheads – the amygdala is to blame.

'This reaction can be imprinted in a developing brain in such a way that it becomes the blueprint for trauma potentially throughout life. That's not to say that everybody who became hysterical at the armed holdup had childhood abuse – it may only be the *perception* of trauma in the child. So a child that's particularly sensitive might perceive trauma where the situation is actually quite benign, like something bad that happened to a character in a storybook.'

Once it's imprinted, though, it becomes part of your psychological makeup. Studies have shown abused children detect threats more readily than others and are more primed to react; this part of their brain is simply over-responsive. Like any other muscle, it's bulging from the constant workouts. But no matter how cosy and sheltered your childhood was, there's a very real chance you were still traumatised by something along the line. Even something as seemingly simple as watching TV with your parents can cause trauma that's scarily real, according to Paul.

'A good example of that is when the Twin Towers went down on 9/11 and the news broadcast updates every five or ten minutes with the footage of the planes crashing into the buildings over and over. There were kids watching it on TV and saying, "Mummy, Mummy – another plane crashed into the building!" Every time they'd see it, it seemed like a different incident because they only had a very primitive brain to work with. It was very distressing for them. It's quite a well-researched and written-up example of that kind of vicarious trauma.'

So the way you deal with trauma: you have your childhood to thank for that. But since we're not tots any more, what we now have to do is figure out how to deal with any fresh hell that comes our way. And there are two ways to do that – you either make it part of your new normal or you separate it as that god-awful thing you will probably never come to terms with but have to accept happened nonetheless. This goes for everything – EVERYTHING – you find tough about life and what it throws at you.

'It's a decision point in therapy in terms of if we aim for getting over it or whether we aim for getting past it,' says Paul. 'So in every therapeutic context, the decision is made between the integrative pathway and the dissociative pathway, if you like. The integrative pathway brings the trauma into your world view, and you try to understand it and make sense of it – then resolve it as being an integral part of your life. Then the dissociative pathway is where you consider it's not possible to come to terms with it. It's just that hard a trauma you can't reconcile it with your world view. So the decision then is to go down the pathway towards managing it as part of your life and not letting it have too much of a consequence on your present and future.'

For example, maybe you've just had a breakup. I've personally had more of these in my time than Steve Irwin had khaki shorts and dealt with a bunch more in my decade as a columnist for *Cosmopolitan*. In that moment, when you're on the receiving end of it, there is nothing in the world more traumatic than a breakup. It's an absolutely wrenching thing. However, as a general rule, you will eventually get over it. You will find someone else. You will live to love again. It doesn't feel like it at the time, but you know somewhere in your gut when people say those things to make you feel better, they're right.

Until, that is, they're not right. Until you have that one that scrambles your insides so much you feel like you've been put in a paint separator and left to rattle overnight. It's been eighteen months and you still can't accept it. Two years passes. Five. Coming across their face on social media is like a king hit to the heart. Songs never cease to remind you of them. Sometimes you shed a tear when you think about them. Other times you drink too much so you don't have to.

Yeah, so at this point you might have to admit you're not going to get over this person. Not ever. What I – and Paul – are telling you is *you don't have to*. There's always a second option. You just have to accept they took a gigantic bite out of the cheese wheel of your life and you're not getting that masticated mush back.

Put the memories of that person in a box in your brain marked 'Fragile: do not remove' and know it will be there forever. Visit it when you need to, but not too often, and get on with the parts of your life you can get on with. The cooking, the cleaning, the movies, the kids' birthday parties, the ordering of coffee, the booking of holidays, the shaving of various body parts. Just let that box gather dust while you do it. Eventually it will just become part of the furniture.

You *do* have to stop letting the trauma of the thing run your life, but you don't have to 'get over it'. Not now, not ever. Yes, you broke up. Yes, that person died. Yes, you got cancer. Yes, you got fired. It happened and it won't un-happen. You can't change what's transpired; you can only change what happens next. It will always be there, that thing, like a malignant elephant in your headroom. But if you can get to a point where it only affects ninety-nine per cent of your day instead of one hundred, then ninety-five per cent instead of ninety-nine, then ninety instead of ... (you catch my sports ball), then you're golden. You're more than golden – you're a living, breathing, functioning human being who's making progress.

We've been taught by pop culture that dissociating from an event isn't ideal. In fact, you've probably heard the word 'dissociate' used negatively in several serial-killer movies and at least one flashback drama starring Nicolas Cage. But for some people, 'getting over it' simply isn't possible – and you might just be one of these people.

In some cases, 'not getting over' your trauma is something people can understand, like, say, in the case of the death of a child. Other times, it might be something people struggle to empathise with, like that time you over-plucked your eyebrows. But despite the criticism, Paul maintains it's a valid approach. And he has a pretty stark example.

'When our service people returned from the Second World War, we didn't have great counselling facilities at that time. What happened was many people just dissociated. They came back to jobs and families and a life. But they had to manage their traumas from the war by simply putting them on the shelf. Every now and again, perhaps on ANZAC Day, you'll find all the old diggers getting together. They're in the pub, talking about all of the pranks they got up to and the camaraderie and the good times they had. But what they don't talk about is bayoneting people in the killing fields. If you were to suggest to them they did that, they'd tell you it was ridiculous. They've dissociated from that period of their lives. Every so often, they might have a relapse into a temper tantrum or even depression. But generally speaking, they've actually managed their lives pretty well by having put the trauma on the shelf or dissociating from it.

'Conversely, when the Vietnam vets came back home, we had a much more enlightened counselling facility. So we embarked upon the process of trying to integrate these experiences they had during the war. And it's a long process – a lot of vets have had counselling for forty years now and those experiences are still not integrated. So it's not a case of one being better than the other, necessarily. It just depends on the personality, the style of the trauma, and whether in fact it's a better decision to go dissociative or integrative. In my experience, you provide the kind of treatment that's helpful and don't be too judgemental either morally or ethically about which is better or which is worse.'

What Paul is saying is that it's your job is to develop a relationship with your trauma that works for you. That's what this book is about when it's at home. Resilience isn't about getting over what's happened to you – a lot of the time it's *just getting through it*.

'Again, the Twin Towers coming down makes a significant case for this,' says Paul. 'As a survivor of that, if you were to try to integrate it into your world view, you'd have to believe that it's reasonable for terrorists to deliberately fly planes into tall buildings to kill as many people as they can. That's a hard ask, integrating that. And if that was your world view, that such an act was reasonable, then you'd never go into a tall building again. You'd never go over a foot bridge. You'd never get onto a plane. So it would be unilaterally disastrous for your life. It's much better to decide it was a freak accident, that it's been resolved in terms of security and better strategies, and that people will therefore largely remain safe.'

Whatever's necessary to not have your brain implode in on itself: that's what you do. Seems like a perfectly reasonable coping strategy to me – one that has nothing to do with kale or turmeric or yoga or tea or things that feel utterly useless to you when trauma is a fresh and pulsating wound. This is just getting on with it the only way you can, and if that means cutting the hurt out and putting it out of sight instead of trying to put a bandage on it and nurse it back to health, that's okay.

'It's absolutely not to be discredited, that kind of pathway,' says Paul. 'Another very clear example from my own experience was the bombing of the JW Marriott Hotel in Jakarta in 2003. We found the Indonesian workers were ready to go back to work the next day. And the reason was because there were no safety nets for them – if they didn't work, their families suffered, possibly died. There's no workers comp or accident and injury insurance, or any kind of Medicare or any free hospitalisation or anything. There's none of that. So what they did, collectively, was decide a ghost had infiltrated the hotel and set revenge upon them. Now that was done and the ghost was abated, it was okay to go back to work. Their cultural view helped them to dissociate, which was the only option they had.'

As a person so lazy I'm practically horizontal, I'm personally just peachy with dissociation from a trauma if that's what you need to be your best in this imperfect world. What I – and the rest of humankind – are probably going to be less accepting of, however, is letting that trauma define you from here on out.

'Well, here, again, you're covering some very important points.'

Thanks, Paul – I do my best.

'Some people do allow trauma to define them, to their detriment. They simply hang on to the disaster. One of the fundamental traits of people with PTSD is that they keep their trauma very close to them. It's almost like they're too fearful to look away from it or to not focus on it. Because should they let their guard down, or their vigilance – being the technical term – it may jump up and bite them. So they keep it very close. Often people go on to allow their trauma to define them forever.

'A good example of that was the Port Arthur shootings. Because after that happened, a lot of people refused to get better. The reason for that, of course, was all of the secondary data – this was a unique event in Australian history and we threw everything at it. There were compensations, there were work-cover payments, there were all manner of reminders of it coming up all the time. Some people, when they sense that they might get compensation for something – this is often the case after car accidents as well – they'll linger longer. Then the trauma does start to define them. We're still treating people after Port Arthur twenty and then some years later. Because while they remain sick, they're not forgotten. They're given sympathy. They're acknowledged and oftentimes compensated, psychologically.'

This is something we've all done to some degree. Letting our boss give us more time off than we need or allowing our friends to shower us with free Negronis and mozzarella sticks after a breakup we probably knew deep down was a good idea anyway. Still, even that's probably better than just ignoring an absolute turd of a situation. (Psychologists have a term for that too, of course: the ostrich effect. No prizes for guessing why.)

Essentially trauma is and always will be a complicated hedge maze of dead ends and labyrinthian solves. Most importantly, though, whatever it is: it matters. There's nothing too small not to be traumatic. 'If it worries you, it worries you,' says Paul. And if the Sheriff of Shockingham says it, you know it's true. Our job now is to get you to a place where you're happy that thing happened to you in the first place. Yes, that's right – I said *happy*.

CHAPTER THREE

Lucky pigs
(Or: How happiness really works)

If trauma is something we want to escape *from*, then unbridled happiness is the thing we want to escape *to*. It's the Bahamas of emotional states and the hormones it releases are those swimming pigs you see on Instagram wading around in the warm Caribbean waters. The whole thing is essentially its own glorious reward.

So what does happiness mean to you?

I'm kidding – we're not going to be *that* book. How very tedious. Much like trauma, the answer to that question is highly personal, so I'm not going to even *try* to tell you what happiness should mean to you. What I can tell you, though, is most people have no idea how happiness works. None.

To start with, did you know we all have a genetically predetermined level of happiness which is responsible for roughly fifty per cent of how 'happy' we are at any given time? A full half of how happy you will ever be is just floating around in your DNA. Considering the pursuit of happiness is arguably humankind's greatest single goal, this little titbit is a rather astounding discovery.

It's also why we should laud scientists and researchers and stop idolising singers and actors, just quietly. This is genuinely, life-changingly important stuff.

This does also mean some people are simply hardwired at a lower set point than others and gravitate towards depression more often than not. If that describes you, that's okay – it's how you're made. Knowing roughly where your set point sits on the spectrum is a solid first step. And there are definitely ways to hack your genes – you too can be the Spiderman of happiness if you get bitten by the right bug. Because while a full half of your joy might be determined by birth, research shows only ten per cent is governed by external circumstances. Which leaves a remarkable forty per cent secured by choice: your choice.

Choosing to be happy isn't like flicking a switch, of course – it's a lifelong practice. Like playing the piano or meditation or parenting. And it's easier for some than for others. But there are ways to make the choice easier – oh, there are ways. What I want to do in this tome is break down the wishy-washy vagueness that so often pervades this kind of discussion and get down to real, operational activities. The ones that don't include ashrams and long-winded journalling. Because those things simply don't work for everyone. And the ambiguity of the advice given in this area is often frustrating to the point of losing faith in the skilled happiness you were seeking in the first place.

For example: 'focusing on the positive' is probably the most parroted piece of advice you'll find in the happiness blogosphere. Once upon a time I found this infinitely useful. No matter what happened to me – whether it was a breakup, getting fired, wrecking my car – I'd trained myself to think, 'Oh well, you know what? At least I don't have cancer!' and then I'd go on my now reasonably merry way. I'd focus on the positive and it worked a treat. For me, remembering what I had to be thankful for was as easy as repeating that one little mantra.

Then of course I actually *got* cancer and my entire mental model went sailing out the window, along with my ponytail and all my bras. In the end, happiness had become a Pavlovian response to not having cancer. Ironic, I know.

Eventually, accepting my much-maligned malignancy meant I had to readjust my framework, which meant reassessing what I had to be thankful for. And it was of course so much more than having or not having cancer. It was my mum and my friends and hot water and sunshine and vibrators and cheese and false eyelashes and dogs. I wanted to squeeze out every bit of the forty per cent of happiness I was psychologically allowed to determine, so I made sure I deemed it pretty fucking amazing to even be alive, actually. Such an odd happenstance, after all, that any of us are. That we can walk and talk and interact like this in a book, one of humankind's best and greatest inventions. What luck!

But this was obviously a mammoth process which involved a lot more than a perky suggestion in a listicle. Someone telling me to 'just focus on the positive' was about as far from the reality of how I got to that point as could be. For me, getting cancer was the thing that made me realise resilience isn't like jumping on a trampoline. It isn't about ups and downs and bouncing back. It just becomes a way of life. One entirely based on our own uncomfortable, harrowing, inevitable trauma.

Research tells me this is true, and we've had an inkling about it for quite a while. Back in the '60s in fact, a psychologist named Victor Goertzel discovered that three quarters of the famous and successful faces he studied (people like Frida Kahlo and John D Rockefeller) were people who had come from troubled backgrounds. These weren't people who had rebounded from a perceived slight – they'd had ongoing, systemic adversity in their lives and dealing with it became part of their world view. Resilience became a constant. And that resilience bore prosperity like a dairy cow giving birth – all noisy, all messy, all unapologetic, all the time.

Of course, having to be tenacious against a world which is trying to beat you down is obviously not an ideal situation. I'm certainly not suggesting you go out and get yourself an alcoholic partner or a round of domestic abuse so you can toughen up. In fact, I don't suggest those things at all, ever. But when you do find yourself in such a mire, it can seem like there's no end in sight. Trying to 'just be positive' when you don't know if you'll have a roof over your head next week is like trying to sop up an ocean with a sponge.

Still, the more we learn about trauma, the more we're seeing what it does for our ability to choose when we want to be happy. Here's an example that tickled my particular fancy …

Let me introduce you to Dr Tim Sharp. Tim is the founder of The Happiness Institute, an Australian organisation dedicated to coaching people to joy. I'm aware happiness experts are starting to become more ubiquitous than yoga instructors in some wellness sectors, but there's a couple of key reasons I like Tim for the job. One: he's got three degrees in psychology, including a PhD, so you just know he knows his stuff. And two: Tim also happens to have depression. Surely how a happiness expert deals with depression is a case study inside the eye of the resilience storm.

'For me, depression and happiness are actually quite separate,' he tells me. Quite joyfully too, I might add, which is almost satirical when you think about it.

'My depression comes and goes,' he continues. 'And when it comes, I don't enjoy positive emotions for hours, days or, sometimes, weeks. But I've learned that eventually it will pass. And quite separate to this, I've created and am lucky enough to live a great life. So even when I'm feeling miserable I can still acknowledge that my life is a good one … even if I don't feel good. That being said, suffering quite severe depression has made me appreciate happiness more. It's also helped me empathise with and help others who are suffering … which I then find satisfying, which makes me feel good.'

He's like the human version of a Möbius strip in an endless chicken-or-egg loop of empathy. But then, he's a happiness expert – so I guess he knows his way around an emotional paradox.

'Early on, I saw depression as something to be "fixed" or "cured" or "beaten". A battle to be won! I now know it's not something I'll ever win. But this isn't a negative because my depression brings me some good in a strange way. It helps me understand others, connect with others and it's led me to do some incredibly satisfying work. So now I see it as something to be managed; it's a part of me. Just a part, not all. Don't get me wrong – when I'm depressed, I don't feel happy. But what I can do is remind myself that at some point in the future I will experience happiness again. I don't expect or want to be happy all the time – I just try to do the best I can and I know if I'm diligent with my self-care I'll feel good more often than not. And that's not just good for me, but it's also good for my wife and children, my family and friends, and my colleagues and clients.'

Basically, Tim is the perfect example of how trauma and happiness are two nemeses who secretly need the other to thrive. They're like Holmes and Moriarty, neither quite at their best without the other. Whether you're stricken with depression of the clinical kind or just the occasional social kind, this is worth remembering.

'No one is happy all the time; that would be unhealthy and it would be unrealistic to expect constant joy. Negative emotions – such as anger and frustration, stress and anxiety – are normal and appropriate. But obviously we don't want too much of the unpleasant ones. Finding the right balance of positive to negative emotions is challenging, but we should aim to have at least three times more positive emotions than negative ones if we really want to live our best lives – if we really want to flourish.'

There, you see why I like him? Real, aspirational equations. I like that in an expert.

He's conscientious too: 'This is very important – because although I advocate optimism, it's important to note that optimism differs from "positive thinking" by being grounded in *reality*. It's helpful to focus on the positives, but it's also important to face up to the cold hard realities, whatever they might be, and deal with them as best we can. Knowing failures and setbacks are inevitable – and not all bad – means you can survive being rocked and, more often than not, come out the other side stronger than before.'

Reality is the key word for this whole experiment. What are the most realistic ways to deal with what feels like an almost untenable situation? Because live long enough and you'll find yourself engulfed in one. You probably already have or you wouldn't be here.

I'm not going to be a cockwaffle about positive thinking, mind you – if you've never had it yourself, give the 'at least I don't have cancer' one a try. It's surprisingly effective when your complaints include things like someone stealing your lunch from the office fridge, losing your phone or having a fender bender on the way home.

If we're trying to find something as seemingly elusive as happiness, however, we surely need to quantify it in some way. So how do you measure something so ineffable? Something as intimate as what makes you tick? Actually, there's a whole UN-funded research paper for that ... it's called the World Happiness Report. Apt. And since we need to calibrate happiness in some way, this seems like a good place to start.

The report basically utilises experts from around the world and mashes their expertise together to come up with an equation for how happy an individual country or culture is. The formula takes into account six variables:

- GDP per capita,
- social support,
- healthy life expectancy,
- freedom to make life choices,
- generosity, and
- freedom from corruption.

These hefty-sounding things all boil down to make the soup that is effectively the global happiness scale. At the time of printing, the top five happiest countries in the world of the 156 ranked were Denmark, Switzerland, Iceland, Norway and Finland, in that order. In comparison, Australia, the US and the UK came in at ten, eighteen and nineteen, respectively.

It stands to reason that the happiest countries produce some of the happiest people. So what do these countries have going on that the rest of us don't?

They're certainly not the richest countries in the world. They do, however, have a smaller gap between the rich and the poor than a lot of other countries. So more equality then. They also seem to have low levels of unemployment and high education levels. And their political stability is relatively off the charts. Parental leave levels for men are offered and taken at record highs. Suicide rates are at record lows. Gender equality and sustainability are matters of national importance. They also have shorter working hours than much of the rest of the world.

When I look at these characteristics, what I notice most is that these things have almost nothing to do with individual circumstances and almost everything to do with a society that cares. People who give a fuck about other people, if you like. Which I do.

And that is where most of us get happiness wrong. We treat it like an inside job. As something that comes from within, when it actually has a whole lot to do with what's happening on the outside, with what we're getting from other people.

'Happiness isn't a solo sport,' says Tim. 'One of the strongest findings from the research is: other people matter. That is, good quality relationships are vital for our happiness, health and wellbeing. Relationships allow us to enjoy the good times more and get through the tough times better. Other people help us feel connected and not alone. Plus, happiness isn't just feeling good; it's also doing good, so when we help others we feel good within ourselves at the same time.'

Essentially, the answer doesn't lie in you sitting in a room alone manifesting happiness bubbles from the great beyond.

In other words, don't believe the hype – the universe does not have your back. It's mostly empty space with a few notable gas balls hurtling around inside it. It doesn't have a grand plan it's waiting to unveil to you when you're ready and having a good hair day. It doesn't care about a text you're waiting for and certainly didn't sabotage your job interview because it 'wasn't meant to be'. You probably just fucked it up. Or the interviewer didn't like the shoes you were wearing. Human beings are flawed like that. The universe is really under no obligation to help you out. But while it mightn't care so much, you'll find your allies do. So hitch your wagon to people, not macrocosms. You never know when the cheese is going to fall off your proverbial cracker – and you're going to need some friends when it does. Because happiness, as we've seen, does actually come from the outside as much, if not more, as it comes from the inside.

Just don't get external happiness confused with external affectations, because that's a whole other Band-Aid you don't need. 'Treat yo'self' has become such a common catchcry, it's easy to seek temporary solace in the purchase of a bar of chocolate or a new pair of shoes. I certainly did when I was first diagnosed with cancer, only it was expensive headscarfs and calorific doughnuts that I chose to lean into.

But did it help? It did not. Because happiness – however temporary – really doesn't come from extravagance; it comes from things far less frivolous.

'Western society has increasingly become a very materialistic and consumerist society,' says Tim. 'That's not entirely bad, but the research clearly shows that more and more "things" won't make us happier and happier. In fact, the minimalist movement is gaining so much favour because many of us are learning that less is sometimes more. This doesn't mean we can't ever enjoy a new purchase, but it does mean if we're thinking of buying something new, we should ask ourselves whether or not it's going to really add value to our lives.'

So if you want to treat yourself, I suggest you do it by letting go of the supposition that the universe is going to provide for you like an invisible destiny-giving unicorn that's been secretly watching your every move since birth, and instead work on furnishing your own future.

'Most experts now agree that happiness can be sought and created, but more so as a consequence of engaging in healthy and helpful behaviours. It can be both a destination and the journey. But it most definitely requires being clear about priorities – because what's just as important as determining what we need to do to live better lives is determining what we *don't* need to do. Whether it's watching the news or going to every party or buying everything we're advertised. If we define it clearly, in our own terms, it need not be intangible. This is something not enough people do! In fact, I'd go so far as saying that if we don't define what happiness means for us, we'll never enjoy as much of it as we could.'

You hear that? Define your priorities and you'll be more likely to be happy even when you're not. Another emotional paradox that's far more rooted in reality than 'thinking happy thoughts'.

Sonja Lyubomirsky – one of those UN-sanctioned experts from the World Happiness Report who basically came up with the whole 50/40/10 theory and has written several books on the subject (one with its own theme song) – has done more research on this matter than most. Her studies show that this type of happiness – the type that is not directly related to a person's circumstances, but driven by that person's behaviours and reactions – has long-lasting consequences. Things like higher incomes, longer marriages and a better immune system.

'I have always been struck by the capacity of some individuals to be remarkably happy, even in the face of stress, trauma or adversity,' she says on her website. 'My students and I have found that truly happy individuals construe life events and daily situations in ways that seem to maintain their happiness, while unhappy individuals construe experiences in ways that seem to reinforce unhappiness.'

So you see, the goal is less about achieving some kind of nirvana and more about shifting the way you view the world. Reframe how you see your situation and you stop setting yourself up for failure and start living in a far more optimistic capacity.

'Another way of thinking about it is that happiness is feeling good, but it's also about being satisfied with our lives overall – even if we're not necessarily feeling great within the moment,' says Tim. 'It does come naturally to some people, but not to everyone. At the same time, it's worth noting for those it doesn't come easily to, it can be learned. And just like learning any other skills, we can become better at happiness if we practise the right sorts of strategies. And the practice required is simply a matter of asking ourselves questions such as: Is there any good to be found in this situation? How can I deal with it? Is there anything I can learn from this? If it's bad, will it last forever?'

Ask and ye shall receive.

But if you're in a rut so deep you feel like your DNA-driven fifty per cent is letting you down and your circumstantial ten per cent is heavy enough to squash that flighty forty per cent entirely, you're far from alone. And at those times questions hardly feel ample enough to make a dent. It's far too easy to find yourself asking other, far less helpful questions like: Why me? What did I do to deserve this? When am I going to catch a break?

So instead of trying to just wrestle with that forty per cent over the coming chapters, I want to work out how to hack the whole enchilada, DNA and all. Don't worry – I have oodles of experts on my side.

'Choice is almost certainly more than that forty per cent in some ways,' says Tim. 'Because the choices we make can change our circumstances and even the way our genes express themselves.'

Good news for those of us who aren't the Dalai Lama.

But before we can get to that, we have to deal with what's already making us unhappy. The unfortunate agony of living, if you will. The acceptance of the shit sandwich you're in, with pain behind you and pain in front of you. I'm not trying to be defeatist – far from it. Pain is just a natural byproduct of being alive. The trick to being happy through all of it, though, is resilience. And that only comes after we are able to look pain right in its ugly little face and say, 'Thank you, friend.'

How do we do that?

We learn to love pain for the guru it is.

Because in the end, I promise you're going to be okay if:

- You're alive.
- You want to be okay.

That's basically it. Congratulations on your decision to be okay. You win at life. Celebrate with a friend. The rest is gravy.

Okay, granted it's a thick, viscous gravy a lot of people drown in … but turn the page and I'll teach you how to rise above all the icky froth and make the most of that forty magnificent per cent on the other side.

CHAPTER FOUR

It was *Planet of the Apes*

(Or: The upside of pain)

The first day I totally understood loss – like, hurts-in-the-chest loss – went a little something like this ...

'Did you understand what the doctor said?'

This was my mother talking to my father.

He rolled his head to the side to look up at her.

'He said it's time to go.'

In this moment, it felt like I had walked in on my parents having sex. Something I never actually did, thank gods. But it struck me as an epic intrusion of intimacy. Like I'd accidentally encroached on a moment only two people who have shared their whole lives together can understand and appreciate. A moment that's not meant for anyone else. Not even their daughter.

It would be a matter of hours, maybe days, the doctors said.

And so the vigil began.

As we sat together – my parents, my sisters and I – no one really knew what we were supposed to be doing. We paced, we watched clocks, we stifled sniffles. Almost every half an hour someone would run down to the cafeteria for coffees and KitKats. Only no one actually ate the KitKats, so they just kept piling up. My father had stopped eating entirely by this point, so it was an odd juxtaposition to see him propped up next to a Jenga-like tower of chocolate and wafers.

We stayed in that hospital room for four days. Each taking shifts staying awake, sleeping in the big chair, sleeping on the floor.

It's fair to say our society doesn't deal well with the true toll of death as it exists in the making of. We've lost the art of grieving someone while they're still alive; we've sugar-coated it so that it's more of a postscript and less of a process. But few deaths are actually instantaneous and so we're stuck in this mollified limbo where everyone feels at a loss. It's heartbreaking.

By the end of the fourth day, everyone but my dad and me was dozing. The TV was on, but I paid little attention to it. Instead, I sat and watched my father breathing. The very act seemed laborious for him and, even though there was nothing I could do, I hovered over him like a purposeful mosquito.

Eventually I felt the need to fill the silence that had surrounded us for so long. It was midnight, after all – the witching hour – and hospitals are eerie after midnight.

'This is such a great story, huh?' I said.

I was talking about the late-night film that had just started and was clearly intended to fill the space between *The Late Show* that had just finished and the breakfast television which was to come. Even though we'd watched this movie half a dozen or more times before – it was one of his favourites – I just needed something to say. I turned back to look at the glowing box, not expecting a response. He hadn't spoken in hours. Just *being* looked painful, let alone the effort of trying to push words out.

'It is what it is,' he replied calmly.

My head snapped back, a look of surprise no doubt etched on my puffy, tear-stained face. I was so taken aback I couldn't even think of anything with which to counter. I knew he wasn't talking about the film, of course, but about life in general. He'd said it many times before, in fact, but it had never seemed as stoic. And it had certainly never seemed as effortful. I'm not sure if he knew it would come to pass at the time, but those were the last words he ever said. He died before the movie finished.

In hindsight, this was probably one of the most defining moments of my life. Not because that was his last utterance, as seemingly poignant as it was, but because of what he meant when he said it. This was something that took me quite some time to figure out. In the moment, I had thought it was sad and heart-rending and maybe even a little aloof – but I didn't realise until much later just how much, if you mean it, that sentence can shape your reaction to almost anything.

As long as you mean it.

The revelation came years later – not long after I'd had my own tumour suspicions confirmed. The thing is, the weeks after a cancer diagnosis are weird. Like, mind-numbingly weird. Just as with anything tragic that happens in your life – the death of a loved one, the loss of a limb, a terminal illness – it takes a while before it becomes a thread you're willing to weave into your tapestry. But eventually you have to, otherwise you become a shell of a person and there's far too much life to be had in too short a time to resign yourself to being a husk.

But you often don't react straightaway; it takes some time. You float through life with the world turned sideways for a while, just percolating facts until such time as your brain decides what its next move will be. For me, that time came the day I started chemotherapy – two years to the day my own father had died from his last-ditch, Hail Mary round of chemo. That was the day it clicked for me: he was right. I knew what he meant. What he *really* meant when he said those words in that hospital bed. It really *is* what it is. No more, no less. Time is linear, it doesn't go backwards – at least not yet. So what has happened has happened, and the sooner you stop feeling hard done by and move forward, the better. Even if what you're moving forward into is death.

This is a concept that isn't without controversy – *it is what it is* is often described as meaningless, irrelevant, rhetorical. But for me it was the seed of an epiphany that helped me realise I was going to be okay. That I could choose to green-light the buoyancy of this experience.

For whatever reason, I already had it in me to make the choice to react like this. And it's going to look and feel slightly different to you. But once you can get to 'it is what it is', life – and death – get significantly easier.

The day I realised that was honestly the day I started being really, truly happy. Sure, it's a wee bit dramatic that it happened the day I first sat in a chemo chair, but that's just where my life story had plopped me. Yours will be somewhere else, thinking of someone else, pondering an entirely different future. But if you can toggle that switch, you'll get there too. There's a little button in our brain, I think, that gets turned off when we're about three or four and tends to remain dormant for the rest of our lives. It controls our ability to not give a fuck what anybody else thinks or does. For a child, that might mean something as simple as wearing a tutu with gumboots. For an adult, it tends to mean a lot more. But if you can manage to switch it back on again, it will give you an immeasurable aptitude for getting on with it. For being happy about stupidly Lilliputian things like a snip of sunshine or sand in your butt crack. Real Disney-type shit. Because while pain is inescapable in this life, suffering is not. And pain, as it turns out, can actually be quite useful.

Let me ask you a question: what's your first memory? Because for a reasonable number of people, it's a traumatic one. Not because everyone's going around having horrific childhoods, but because those are the memories that stick. Mine is of having eight stitches put in my chin after falling off some play equipment at day care. Which, at three years of age, was the most daunting thing I had ever experienced. I can remember the dress I was wearing, the colours of the mural in the children's ward, even the taste of the strawberry ice cream I got to placate me afterwards. It, and the scar, stick with me until this day.

Research shows that around a quarter of people have similarly traumatic first memories. They linger because of the emotion attached to them. The sheer novelty. I had an otherwise very mundane and trauma-free childhood for the most part, but that one memory stands out like a neon billboard in a sea of handwritten garage sale signs. It was the first time I realised the world wasn't always going to go the way I wanted it to and that some things were going to hurt. It was also the first time I realised wailing a lot gets you ice cream, but that's a different story.

Whether you have an analogous tale or not, we all eventually realise this kind of pain is inevitable. It's as much a part of the human experience as love or curiosity or fear. So how it is useful?

In almost every way.

Toddlers, for example, learn pretty swiftly that touching a hot stove leads to hurt. Teenagers quickly glean the same thing about tequila. Pain is the fastest and most effective learning process there is.

We even learn to rate our discomfort in a 'better the devil you know' sort of way, as a tool to cognitively get through the day.

Will the pain of having my boss mad at me for missing that big presentation outweigh the pain of having to go to work with the flu? Will the pain of having a four-year-old jump on me at 6 am when I have a hangover be greater than the pain of telling my friends I can't meet them for drinks now? Will having to pay for new tyres today be more painful than having to wait for roadside assistance when one blows in six months' time?

We're all just living, breathing computers constantly making decisions that lead us to the best possible outcome. The one that comes with the least amount of perceived pain.

But why do some people seem to thrive in times of stress while others fall apart like a house of cards built on a fault line?

I like to think it's essentially a great big emotional version of a process called hormesis. Hormesis happens in all kinds of life forms, big and small, and is a natty little biological mechanism whereby a beneficial effect comes from low-dose exposure to a toxin that said life form would otherwise find intolerable.

Would you like the non PhD version? What doesn't kill you makes you stronger.

Full disclosure here: the term hormesis is typically only used by toxicologists to describe the effect of things like radiation and other biohazards, but I actually think it's pretty easily transferrable to emotions. Some people just happen to go through huge periods of personal growth when they go through something traumatic. It's an adaptation to stress; a trick of their biology. But if you don't naturally flourish under stress, can you learn from this process? Is there a hormesis class you can take? A pill? What if you kill a hormetic person during a full moon and drink their blood? There has to be a way.

Well, you can learn, as it happens. It's like lifting weights – the first time you do it, it's hard and painful. But your muscles learn to adapt. You become bigger, better, stronger. You've probably been practising your whole life and not even realised it.

Let me put it this way – remember your first breakup? Your first *real* breakup? You probably sobbed a lot, drove past their house a few times, maybe even begged them for another chance? By the time you go through your fourth or fifth relationship breakdown, though, you might cry them a river, but you tend to forgo the drama after a while and skip straight to the vino and fuck-'em party. Your heart, for better or worse, has some scar tissue now and you know the drill. You'll have setbacks, of course, but there's no breakup like that first breakup.

And here's why that first one is so hard: we fall in love with the idea rather than the reality. The reality is that very few people spend their entire lives with the first person they date. And there's a reason for that – the person you are when you're sixteen is decidedly different to the one you are when you're twenty-six, thirty-six or forty-six. You've got growing and travelling to do, mistakes to make and people to have informative, revealing sex with. You need to experience a lot of life before you're comfortable enough with who you are not to lose yourself in another person.

I remember my first bone-shattering breakup well – his name was Wes and I drove past his house at least three times in the space of a single weekend. Once I even had to make a quick getaway after I was spotted by his mum, who was in the driveway hauling groceries in from her car. Awkward.

I was seventeen and, considering I thought my world was over at the time, it's telling that almost twenty years later I can't even remember his last name. But breakups almost always involve mourning the idea of the life you thought you were going to have with someone. Not the person themselves, but the world you created with them in your head. This head-partner is generally kinder and richer than the original and almost certainly never turns down sex. They look good holding your children and maybe even squeeze out tears of joy when you walk down the imaginary head-aisle. And this isn't just true of falling head over Converse All-Stars for the idea of a person, but also a job, a holiday, a car or losing the last five kilos. Anything you want so bad you can feel it in your marrow.

What we need to get past all these types of pain is grit. Hormesis-induced mental grit. The type of resilience you can only learn from exposure to adversity. So how do you get it? Let me hand you over to a man named Ben Newman.

Ben is essentially Tony Robbins meets Coach Taylor and he's in the business of mental toughness. That's genuinely all he does. He speaks on it, he writes about it, he trains other people on how to get it. This is something he's done for the likes of the United States Army, Microsoft, international banks, universities and more professional sports teams than most people could list in a pinch. But here's why I like him – he says stuff like this:

You always have control over the only thing that matters: yourself.

Which is both very true and very hard to digest at the same time. Depending on what you're going through, it can be very easy to react to that with 'Screw you, Ben – your husband didn't leave you for a women half his age and abandon you with three kids and a mortgage, did he?! Take that control and shove it in your pizza hole.'

But he's right. Learning how to control your reaction to things is the smoothest and fastest way to happiness I know. Because suffering is not an inevitable appendage of pain; it's more like a hat we insist on wearing. It's simply a response to stimuli and only you can choose how you respond to something.

'There's a good buddy of mine,' Ben starts telling me when I express my thoughts on this. 'He's a Navy SEAL. And I really like the Navy SEAL's mantra for this. It's simply: "You can bitch about anything for five minutes, but after that you'd better get on with it 'cause people are going to die.'"

Yeah, that sounds like something a Navy SEAL would say.

'And obviously everyone's situation is different. If you're experiencing cancer treatment, that period is going to take more than five minutes. But you need to put a timeline on it. We don't want you to live in La La Land – it's not all unicorns and rainbows – but the reality is for people to complain about most things for more than five minutes is a colossal waste of time.'

As someone who once spent six months asking all my friends, 'Why do you think he broke up with me? No but, like, really?' I'd have to agree with that assessment. It's not to say the pain doesn't last longer and the scars even longer than that, but indulging your pain for too long is most definitely detrimental to your mental grit.

Pain comes in many guises, of course, but let's just gather them all up into one big ball like unwanted slivers of soap. Physical pain is arguably very different from emotional pain, but they are often connected. And they feed off each other in the strangest of ways. Both kinds of pain also come in two varieties, however: temporary and chronic. And the temporary kind is almost certainly getting in your way with unnecessary force.

'Too often people allow their feelings to dictate how they show up,' says Ben. 'So yesterday was a bad day and as a result of yesterday being a bad day, I don't feel like putting myself through it today. Or, on the contrary, because yesterday was so great I'm just going to take today off.'

I don't know about you, but that's how I've lived most of my life. Guilty as charged. But teaching people *not* to do that is a big part of Ben's MO.

'I think people can only truly perform at their highest level when they start giving it their best *one day at a time*.'

Which is something you figure out how to do almost by osmosis when you find yourself in a pickle, like being diagnosed with a degenerative disease or learning to live without someone you once thought of as a limb. But wouldn't it be better to learn how to do it long before you need it to survive? Let me tell you a fun story about the North Dakota State Bison football team to show you what that looks like.

It's okay, I didn't know who they were either.

They happen to be an unusually successful American college football team. At the time of writing, they've won six out of the last seven national championships in division-one college football. Guess who their performance coach is? That's right – it's Ben.

'You'll love this,' he tells me. 'These players aren't allowed to come into the weights room wearing any T-shirts or clothing that have anything to do with a past national championship. The coaches won't allow it. You can't wear any gear that doesn't have to do with winning *that day*. And the message here is "raise the bar". Because I think when people have achieved a high level of success or think they're at the top, they can either be seduced by that success and settle in that dominant position or they can say, "All right, if there's nobody above me I'd better find more within myself. I need to redefine what winning looks like. I need to give a little more." A lot of people win one championship and then never win another one and the reason for that is they continue to define themselves by the last one.'

So basically: if you're not indulging pain for more than five minutes, you shouldn't indulge pleasure for too long either. Because both things can be equally useful in determining future happiness if you let them be educational, rather than sentimental. It might sound a little cold, but when you even these things out what you're left with is a more constant state of contentment, as opposed to fluctuations that can leave you reeling and even incapacitated. You set yourself up for a far more fulfilling everyday if you take each one on its merits, not its laurels.

'The former quarterback of the Bisons is a guy named Carson Wentz, who's now quarterback for the Philadelphia Eagles, who just won the Super Bowl,' continues Ben. 'So when you talk about coming from a culture of success, that's up there. But the manner in which, and the reason why, he's been able to continue to win is because he doesn't define himself by past success. He focuses on winning one day at a time.'

It sounds like sportsball rhetoric, of course: 'winning one day at a time'. But if someone can train themselves not to wallow in success – something I imagine would be rather gratifying – then surely we can also train ourselves not to wallow in the reverse. Which is far less gratifying and therefore an infinitely more worthwhile pursuit.

While this all theoretically works with temporary setbacks, chronic pain is a whole different trawler of sea bass. If temporary pain is a blip, chronic pain is a broken car alarm. It's there, it's awful, it wants your attention and there's nothing you can do about it. This is where mental grit really comes into its own.

'Grit to me is continuing to fight through whatever pain or challenge comes to you,' says Ben. 'It's a series of monotonous behaviours performed over and over and over and over again.'

Which is an interesting way to put it: monotony. When you think of someone with grit, you don't think about what it took to get them there as much as you're impressed by the fact they seem to intrinsically have it together. But of course it was indubitably repetition, not fate, that performed in their favour and got them to that point in the first place.

'You have a choice – I'm going to be fearful and I'm going to quit, or I'm going to have faith that if I work hard and continue these monotonous behaviours over and over and over again, I'm going to get through this. It might take me a little longer, I might experience pain, I might experience challenges, but I'm going to grow through this.'

A lot of the time the way we respond to things feels innate – it's just something in your genetic makeup that means you get jealous when your friend gets a great haircut or irrationally upset when someone doesn't like your cooking. But often, it's a choice. And choosing not to suffer is choosing the most incredible freedom you can imagine.

It works the other way too. For a lot of people walking this planet, their chronic pain comes from the feeling that life hasn't given them a fair suck of the sauce bottle. Their choice is to believe that.

'It becomes a cop-out when people say, "Well, sure, look at these people who have money, of course they're successful." They're doing this because they have guilt which comes from not living their best life and so they start throwing stones at people who are working hard. I always encourage people to stay in their lane – so identify your purpose, your passion, identify what success means to you and fight like hell every single day to achieve that success. I think far too often what happens is people start looking over at what people in the next lane are doing. Why does somebody else have to define your success? I think the critical manoeuvre is when you define what your success looks like.'

But here's the thing about success and happiness … it very rarely has anything to do with what you do for a living. Success could actually be as simple as a room with a view. Having been stuck in a hospital room wondering if I would ever see the ocean again makes me really, really appreciate bodies of water now. A sea, a lake, a puddle on the footpath – it doesn't matter the size or the depth or the clarity. Every time I see one now, I take a really deep breath in and remember the world is a glorious place. I feel successful just being here.

I admit, sometimes these things can get a little too motivational bootcamp, even for me. Pep talks are great, but I like some action to go with my rally cry. I want to go next level. So I asked what the performance coach's performance coach taught him that really stuck. Might as well get meta on this thing, right?

'So my current coach – and I'll never forget this – taught me one of the greatest lessons I've ever learned. It was 2009 and I was doing the planning for my first-ever bootcamp.'

See? Bootcamps, they're a thing.

'This particular year it was in Vegas. So I sent my coach my slides for my presentation. And I had a slide titled "Dream Board".'

Even Oprah had one in 2009; they were all the rage.

'And she said, "That's not the right title." And I said, "What do you mean? It was on *Oprah*: Dream Board. So that's the right title." And she goes, "It should be called a Reality Board. Isn't it more powerful if you call it a Reality Board? It's not your reality yet, but it's going to be." And so I started teaching that concept. Because she was right – when you have the belief that it's going to be a reality, it drives your actions.'

And what is your proposed future reality if not your very purpose? So ... how exactly do we figure out what that is, Ben?

'I think far too many people base their purpose on what somebody else would want for them rather than what drives them. How could you possibly take the necessary action or know what it truly means to operate from your gut if you're doing it for somebody else's idea of success? You need to make an "I am" statement: a statement of belief around achieving something that you believe you can do before it actually happens. Normally when someone asks the question "Who are you?", you give an answer based upon things you've achieved in the past. But what if you answered based on the things you're going to do? What if you said, "I'm Emma and I'm going to be an international bestseller"?'

From your mouth to the ears of the *New York Times* books editor, Ben.

'Okay, but imagine what happens to your daily actions if you wake up thinking, "I'm a *New York Times* bestselling author." When people connect to something they haven't achieved yet, it's followed by the action and the belief that it takes to achieve that thing. And even if it doesn't happen, you can look in the mirror and say, "I gave it my very best." And that's all this is about. Giving your best.'

Let's just outline what we've laid down here.

- Pain is inevitable
- You're probably going through some right now
- You're probably suffering through it, in fact
- But that makes sense because you've basically been traumatised since you were born
- You've already learned a lot from that process, though
- And the rest is a choice.

The choosing, though – that's hard. But one thing I know from personal experience is that when things are too easy, they lose their value. In the same way it's hard to appreciate something you get for free. Even if it's, say, a sample of yoghurt at the supermarket. It simply doesn't taste as sweet as the yoghurt you deemed worthy of spending your hard-earned dollars on.

So let's work on that. Soon I'll have you choosing contentment the way you choose your socks in the morning. But first, we have to get through the grieving period – because all trauma comes with grief. And it's how we handle that grief that sets us up for resilience, which is the happiness springboard I'm here for.

But before we get to that, I just want you to answer one question: what's the most impressive thing that happened in 2010?

If you said the affair between Colin Farrell and Elizabeth Taylor you'd be close. But no. Dig into Chapter Five and the answer will greet you.

Atomic number 117

(Or: How to get through grief)

If I were to casually mention Russia and the US in the same breath, it's not out of the realms of possibility to think of political tampering, the space race or, to a lesser extent, mail-order brides. There's also that pesky purchase of Alaska thing in 1867, which I'm guessing Russia is still slightly stinging from. It's a tumultuous relationship, in any event.

But back in 2010, a group of Russian and American scientists working together for the greater good did something rather mind-boggling ... something you probably never even heard a whisper about.

They invented a new element.

Like a sits-in-the-periodic-table, atomic-weight-having element.

By putting those fancy brains of theirs together and bombarding calcium with berkelium in one of those giant atom-smashing fusion machines scientists get so excited about, a brand spanking new element was born.

It's called tennessine, only fifteen atoms of it have ever been made, and it's the second heaviest substance in our known universe.

With currently no practical application whatsoever, it strikes me as an achievement on par with climbing Mount Everest ... we did it because we could.

Which brings me to a man named Christopher Hall.

Chris didn't have anything to do with tennessine – he's not Russian or American, and to be honest probably doesn't even own a beaker. He lives in Melbourne, Australia and he's the CEO of the Australian Centre for Grief and Bereavement. An organisation whose monthly newsletter is called *The Grief Brief* by the way – don't tell me bereavement counsellors don't have a sense of humour.

Chris has spent decades as a psychologist counselling people on death and loss. He's even a member of the International Work Group of Death, Dying and Bereavement. Did you even know that was a thing? Me neither. But death is obviously a very necessary part of life so it makes sense there would be quite the global industry revolving around it.

When I first stumbled upon Chris, I don't mind telling you I wondered what kind of man he would be. What sort of person dedicates his life to death? How did he end up there and what did he like so much about it? More importantly, was he just a sociopathic Dexter type, fascinated by misery and intent on being part of it? Was he going to be creepy beyond all belief? Should I update my life insurance before gracing his door?

As it turns out, he's the happiest man I've ever met.

It took me days to work out what his deal was. How was he so upbeat when he was surrounded by nothing but agony? Did he feed on death and despair? Was he an actual metamorphic hellhound, somehow escaped from below only to set up shop in a cosy suburb on Australia's pristine coast? But then it snapped – like an airplane seat belt complete with that really satisfying click. I realised it was because Chris was essentially working with the emotional version of tennessine. Just rolling this overwhelmingly heavy thing no one knows what to do with around in his palms. And just like important atom-smashing work, engaging with grief had given him a sense of purpose.

These two things – atom-smashing and grief-counselling – are equally meaningful to the human experience and the expansion of human knowledge. One strives to further science and the other spirituality, but both are trying to make something out of nothing. The only difference is Chris is actually coming up with some answers.

'I'm naturally curious about things, always have been, and I'd often get into trouble for taking things apart and not being able to put them back together again when I was young,' he says. 'I think also for me it was partly about, as a kid, asking difficult questions. My father was actually an Anglican minister, so I grew up immersed in death – I'd look out my bedroom window and see a hearse rock up, or pick up the phone and find a bereaved widow or widower on the other end of it wanting to talk to my dad. Then a significant thing happened when I was eleven, just after I started at a new school. Within a couple of weeks, a teacher came into the room on a Monday morning and said, "Ashley won't be coming back to school." I subsequently discovered that he'd been electrocuted and died at the weekend, only nothing more was said about it. I thought, "Wow, what is it about this that's so unspeakable?"

'Subsequently I did psychology, I worked as a school counsellor and then progressed through education. Now I've been in this job for twenty-one years and it's the most fantastic work. I don't wanna get schmaltzy about it, but it really feels like a calling. And when people say, "Oh my god, how depressing. How could you do a job like that for so long?", I say, "Well, it's a really privileged position because effectively what I spend much of my time doing is listening to love stories."'

Hold up ... love stories?

'Absolutely – grief is the price we pay for love.'

That is PROFOUND, Chris. Please continue.

'When you see grief and love as the opposite sides of the same coin, often what grief is, is love with nowhere to go.'

As much as I loathe them, I think Chris should have his own motivational quote account on Instagram. Agreed? Agreed.

'In terms of bereavement, what we often ask the client to do in the first few sessions is to introduce us to the person who's died in the same way they might introduce us to somebody at a party. In a sense, we can't understand the bereaved person until we get to know the person who died and what that relationship is. So there's lots of storytelling about who this person was. While that often involves stories about the nature of the death and how the person died, it's also the story of how these two met and the love they brought to each other's lives.'

Such an awfully lovely way to talk about grief, wouldn't you say? But it's not easy, inviting death in. Grief doesn't *become* anyone. It's ugly and awkward and heavy-handed. It's often so immense you can't even make out its edges. You're adrift and at the complete mercy of its whims. People who have sailed the same ocean will tell you they've weathered the same storms and that there's a way out. But when every wave is different, how do they know? Maybe you'll be the one to drown where they were rescued?

'Around eight to nine per cent of the bereaved population get into some difficulty,' says Chris. 'Most people respond to losses, incredible losses, incredibly well, but for some people, that process gets derailed. I'd say most of the problems bereaved people have are social problems. It's the inability or the unwillingness of their community to care for them. People move away rather than towards somebody, and that's our own stuff about not knowing what to say. So many people come into counselling, saying, "I'm here because my friends and family have had a gutful of talking about this. I should be over it by now." I think a lot of the models about grief haven't served us well. We can go back to 1969 and Elisabeth Kübler-Ross – many people know her from her work on the five stages of grief: denial, anger, bargaining, depression and acceptance. But the reality is there's no evidence that supports that idea. We're seduced by the simplicity of these sorts of models, by the idea that we can squeeze all human beings into them. It has this emotional promise land of acceptance, but that's just not the way it goes. It's much more complex.

'People see emotions as the gold standard – we need to express our emotions, we need to talk about them, but that's just not always the case. For many people, it's not about wrapping their heart around what's happened, it's about wrapping their *head* around it. It's about making sense of it. We know those who struggle the most are people who are searching for but haven't found any meaning in the experience. It's this life event that remains unmetabolised, unprocessed.'

And this is where trauma comes into it. Your trauma, my trauma. This is why I'll never tell you everything will all make sense one day, when all your planets align and your destiny is fulfilled. Because that's simply not realistic. That, quite frankly, is a little bit dangerous. Because trauma will come for you and not because it was 'meant to be', but simply because things not always going your way is one of the great consequences of being alive. Like Chris says, wrapping your head around that can be one of the most difficult parts of the experience. Life is a beautiful, tangled thing. And sometimes what we're taught can actually be quite counterproductive to living it.

'I think one of the great lies is that time heals all wounds.'

Amen, Chris.

'We know from the research that stuff is not true. When we look at all the factors that influence the intensity of grief, time since the death explains or predicts less than two per cent of stress. Grief therapy is not about saying goodbye or letting go. It's about how do we live, how do we move on from a relationship largely based on somebody's physical presence to a relationship largely based on memory? Grief is a process of relearning the world. The world's a different place and our place in it is different, our relationships are different. Death ends a life, it doesn't end a relationship. We can have complex relationships with living people and we can have complex relationships with dead people. So the absence of someone doesn't mean it's all over, red rover – in fact, it really can just be the beginning in many ways.'

This is where I think it really gets interesting. Because in a lot of ways I think we have grief backwards. We know grief doesn't get easier with time at all – often it's quite the opposite. The longer you're without someone or something, the more you miss them. Each holiday you're without a loved one gets harder; each night out you miss because you're in hospital stings more; each promotion you're passed over for leaves you rawer than the last. Grief can be fresh or stale, but it's forever solid. And unfortunately the longer it's been, the more people whisper, '*It's really time he got over it. It's been years. He needs to move on.*'

We now know that's not how it works, of course. Grief is far more complicated that we generally care to admit. When my dad first passed away, I was stricken but not surprised. He'd been sick for eighteen months, so we knew it was coming. Did that make it any easier to integrate? I doubt it. Anyone who's seen someone wither away to the point of death secretly wishes at least once that they'd died quickly, as in a car accident. And anyone who's had someone ripped away from them suddenly, secretly wishes they'd had eighteen more months with them, even if it meant watching their loved one turn into a wisp of their former selves. It's 'the grass is greener' laced with formaldehyde and toe tags.

Grief is something we usually think of as following death, like an evil rabid puppy. But it's not just death it follows – it's anything that you're having trouble integrating into your normal. It's equally relevant to divorce, breakups, amputations of persons or body parts, and whatever else ails you. Having something that's important to you suddenly withdrawn without your consent is horrific in almost all instances.

'Grief is basically any change,' says Chris. 'Sometimes these seismic changes bring about really significant shifts in people's identity. Mostly they're in positive ways – so we hear people talking about things like not taking life for granted, not putting things off. One of the gifts, then, is perhaps a sense of immediacy. Other times people live in their own private hell because of this social expectation that you'll eventually be fine. When it's a death, we have a funeral. But there aren't many other ways, save perhaps the occasional divorce party, that we come together and acknowledge grief.'

Privately, however, we grieve loss of all kinds. It might be the loss of a friendship, an old life, even a pair of jeans. The most inexplicable grief of all is when you weep for things that haven't even transpired yet. In every breakup, there's the ache of holidays not taken, aisles not walked down and eye-twinkles not realised. These unexpressed loses are often far more upsetting than the thing itself. When you're diagnosed with cancer and are facing your own death, it's the same – the grandchildren not met, books not written and countries not visited. It's mourning the loss of the life you imagined but no longer get to have. That's often the greatest calamity of all. A promise unrealised is tragedy in motion. How beautifully human and flawed is that.

'We tell ourselves stories about the way our lives will play out. These are often described in the literature as "disenfranchised losses", where they're not socially accepted or recognised. They're not seen as meriting attention in the same way. Losing your job is a good example – for many people, career is such a part of who they are. We define ourselves by what we do, we introduce ourselves in terms of what we do. As a bereavement counsellor I've worked with professional athletes who've been delisted for Olympic Games selection – because that loss of professional identity, that's a biggie. But it's not seen as being on the same level as the death of a loved one. The same applies to the death of a pet, or certain relationships that aren't recognised in the same way, such as same-sex relationships in certain areas of society. Even some deaths which evoke anxiety or embarrassment are disenfranchised – we don't talk about the person who died from autoerotic asphyxiation, for example.'

You see why I call this the tennessine of human experience? Heavy.

But by rating grief on a scale like this – where we consider some kinds more important than others – we're doing ourselves a major disservice. And we certainly have some way to go until we can genuinely empathise with each other without judgement – which is incredibly remiss of us, when you think about it. Grief is a universal experience that breaks every class, race and sexual barrier we have. It tears through them with complete and wild abandon. So why can't we talk about it more openly and more freely?

'I think, in many ways, the grief and bereavement field is where sex education was in the 1960s. At least now we can talk about the parts of the human body by their proper names, but I think we're in that place in bereavement where we'll say anything other than "he's dead". That's probably well-intentioned in that people don't want to elicit distress in others, so we use some other euphemism, but these are really problematic. Particularly when you talk about the experience of kids who are told, "I'm so sorry, but Daddy's gone to heaven." Then this kid is in the shed building a ladder to go see Daddy who's up in heaven. It just makes the situation even more complex.'

So in such complicated territory, what's the best way through? We're so sensitive to trauma, yet the idea of being resilient to grief almost makes you seem like an unfeeling monster. But there are ways in which trauma is a superlative teacher, more effective than even time or love. Because sometimes you need to make yourself small in order to see the big picture – and grief has the ability to do that with breathtaking speed and efficiency. So take your trauma for what it is and let it make you feel small and helpless for a while. Because it will – with or without your consent.

'I think fundamentally we can't give grieving people what they want. We can't give them back their baby who's died, we can't give them back their health or whatever else that might be. So that elicits a real powerlessness in a lot of people, because we can't fix you. We live in a culture which is about making things better, but grief is effectively a kind of trauma in itself and as human beings we avoid trauma. We walk away from trauma. It's not about saying to somebody, "Well, look on the bright side," or "It could be worse." I think we're now realising we've underestimated the amount of trauma in bereavement and the amount of loss in trauma.'

Once again: do not let anyone tell you your best friend moving overseas, your cat getting run over or your receding hairline isn't important enough for all of the feels. There's no scale here. But by the same greasy token, do not expect anyone else to be able to understand it, let alone fix it. That's something you have to work out for yourself. Lucky, I suppose, there are plenty of ways in which to do it.

'People will draw upon lots of different frameworks,' says Chris. 'Some might be philosophical, some might be spiritual. We've moved away from cookie-cutter approaches – we know it's highly idiosyncratic and people have different safe places. If you look at spirituality, for example, we often think of spirituality or religion as a scaffold and imagine that people can place their experience on that foundation. In some cases, that's a perfect fit. It's able to hold that experience. Alternatively, though, we see people who place their experience on this scaffold of meaning and it wobbles, it needs to be strengthened. I've counselled people who have said to me they needed to move away from a Sunday School view of God to something more complex, something more nuanced. Other people again might talk about, "How could a loving God allow this to happen?" Their scaffold completely collapses under the weight of their experience.'

That's not to say, of course, you need a god or gods of any kind to get through grief. You obviously do not. In fact, I have a whole new spiritual alternative you might never have considered – more on that later. But the example is sound. Because whatever your thing may be, that mental model that has gotten you through life thus far may not see you through this. What then?

'Grief is a choice-less event, but the way we respond to it is rich in choice,' says Chris. 'So there are lots of things that people can do. And I think that's really exciting. That really anything, if we invest in it with quality, can be grief work. Whether that's gardening, sculpture, listening to music, playing music, reading. We need to think much more broadly about the way that people can be helped and help themselves by engaging in those sorts of things.'

You know what else is great? Honest to goodness great for getting through a shitstorm? Crying in the shower.

'I sometimes think more grieving gets done, or more crying gets done, in showers and swimming pools than in the consulting rooms of bereavement practitioners,' says Chris. 'Because it's a safe place. Many mums have said to me the shower's one of the few places where the kids aren't hassling them and they can actually be completely alone and just sob under the water. Maybe there's something elemental about that, about being in water.'

Agreement from the bereavement big cheese – I'll take that as a win.

But whatever it is that works for you, works for you. You may have to try a lot of different avenues, but when you find it, hold on to it for dear life. And never apologise for what you had to do in order to survive. Unless you kicked the dog or yelled at your partner for burning your grilled cheese, of course; those are things you should apologise for. But not turning up to a party or needing to hog the bathroom – these are things you can forgive yourself for. Everything you need to do when you're grieving is completely perfect in that moment. Death and loss may be inevitable, but somehow it doesn't make them any more expected when they happen to you. The human brain apparently just isn't capable of such a simple equation when emotion is involved. We're just monkeys with car keys.

Other people have been there before you and other people will be there after you. That space between where you are right now and where you want to be: it probably terrifies you, but it will eventually inspire you. And I know exactly how to make that happen. From now on in, each chapter will come with an action. Some are easy, some a little harder. But they are all actual activities you can do to cultivate your resilience. And I'll be frank ... the first one is my absolute favourite.

THINGS YOU CAN DO TODAY

Six things you can do today (or, you know, this weekend, if you're feeling lazy) to help jumpstart your resilience.

CHAPTER SIX

Salt and vinegar chips

(Or: Interrupting your trauma)

The bulging handful of actions I'm about to present to you worked wonders for me, but are all also backed up by science-y types with email sign-offs that look like someone spat up alphabet soup next to their name. Do each of these things and I guarantee you'll feel like a far more robust human by the end of this book. Not in a Dwayne Johnson sense but in a 'I won't break down crying in the supermarket' sense. Which, to be fair, is probably infinitely more useful anyway.

These actions are easy too. Almost laughably so. Not once will you find a step extolling you to 'throw out half your belongings' or a 'take a ten-day meditation retreat'. These are achievable for even the laziest, most sceptical among us. I know because that's me and I did all of them. Just how feasible are they? Well, the first step is to change your underwear.

Actually, I'm getting ahead of myself – the first step is even simpler than that.

Before you wriggle out of your underthings – and I sincerely hope you do – let's talk about what's distressing you. Because it's something, or you wouldn't be sitting here reading this. So the very first thing you have to do is label it.

I know – it sounds like the first step in a really laborious counselling session. On the tedium scale, it's right up there with the question: *'And how did that make you feel?'*

But as a first step in making yourself unfuckwithable, it actually can't be beat.

It works like this …

Step one: choose your word. Actually, you don't even really have to choose it – it's probably already chosen you. This word is a semantic Tupperware container that summaries your trauma. My word was cancer, for obvious reasons. But yours might be divorce, death, bankruptcy, wheelchair, addiction, regret, anxiety, childless, abuse.

Got your word?

Whatever it is, I'm guessing you have some trouble saying it out loud. And here's why: because when trauma is fresh, saying that word opens a door, and a whole squirming, squalid mess of emotion comes tumbling out. Along with tears, more often than not. It's why we all have so much trouble telling people when something traumatic happens. Saying it can feel impossible for days, weeks or even months. After my diagnosis, it took me several days before I could say the word 'cancer' out loud. I would try, but just feel my lip quivering instead. It's a tough word to say, even when you're resilient.

Perhaps your trauma doesn't even feel like one single thing. Maybe it feels more like a person than a thing. Maybe it's hiding behind something else. It's almost always more complicated than it seems at first. Like a David Lynch painting. Or a David Lynch film. Or a David Lynch anything, really.

But labelling your pain is a worthwhile pursuit. So to figure out what's really pressing your buttons, any time you have a new and intense negative feeling overcome you, just do these two things:

1) Pour yourself a large glass of water (or wine, I'm not going to judge – I'd go a shiraz, personally).

2) Sit for ten minutes (put a timer on if you have to), imbibe your beverage and get to work trying to label your wound. If you find yourself feeling particular overwhelmed, change chairs, move rooms – a physical change of space can actually help nudge you into the right mode.

Labelling is a surprisingly helpful assignment. You might be angry but why? Is it because of the actions of someone else, the fact things didn't go as you expected, because something was taken away from you? Just banging around the house being angry isn't going to get you very far. Knowing you're unhappy because you didn't realise how much stock you put into that date going well is more useful. It's then you realise your label is lonely ... which, now that you have it, gives you an excellent place to start.

Labelling your trauma makes it instantly easier to deal with, even if you don't consciously realise it. Just giving your feelings a name means all that turbulent activity going on in your brain shifts straightaway from the emotional section to the thinking section. Quite genuinely, that's a biological thing that happens, which is why psychologists often recommend doing it. Almost immediately you'll have more conscious control of the situation.

It doesn't feel like it initially, mind you. And for a lot of people their label is pretty heavy. Lonely is a good example. It's endemic to your life and hard to change overnight. It's something that isn't easy to lift yourself out of and, in fact, helps dig its own hole. Fixing loneliness isn't as simple as hanging out with a friend. You can be in a room full of people and still feel lonely. So what's the fix when the problem feels more epic than John Farnham's back catalogue?

Ask the world's happiness experts and they all have slightly different ideas on this. But everyone agrees there's no one-size-fits-all strategy. Some people are meditators, some aren't. Some people have success with exercise, some don't. Which is why in this book I'm giving you almost two dozen ways to give it a crack. The likelihood is at least a few will stick with you.

It's also worth remembering unhappiness isn't a disease to be cured. Happiness doesn't exist without it, in fact – and some of the happiest people in the world are those who have been through some of the roughest of times. Through great darkness comes great light and all that.

For other people, such as those for whom the label is bipolar or clinical depression, happiness is less a choice and more a contrariety. If that's you, you'll probably need something a little more pharmaceutical than I can provide, but it's my hope these tactics will still be useful.

It's also more than worth pointing out happiness is statistically abnormal. If you spend a lot of time on social media, it's easy to think otherwise, but most people you run into on a daily basis are somewhere in the middle of the mood spectrum, bobbing up and down and generally just treading water. That, also, is pretty damn human.

The real key to being more mentally robust, more positive and better at not bursting into tears when you break a nail starts with accepting that you're going to have to take it reeeeeal slow. Because the overriding trick is taking tiny little bites. You have to Hansel and Gretel it, going one crumb at a time.

Just like Kyle McDonald.

Kyle is a Canadian blogger who once managed to swap a single paperclip for a house. Not straightaway, of course, but through a series of smaller trades. Trades which included a fish-shaped pen, an empty keg and a recording contract. Kyle is a guy who knows how to take tiny little bites. Take it slow. Be unhurried in the pursuit of a goal.

You need to think of your positive mindset as being like Kyle's house. The mindset is the goal, but you might be led in some odd directions on the way. Don't rush it. Don't expect radical leaps. Enjoy the process. Be open to fish-shaped writing implements and other curios that don't appear to have anything to do with the goal at hand. Be like Kyle.

The easiest way to spark some change is by poking a hole in the membrane of your life. Because at the moment you're encapsulated by it, that membrane, and you could potentially be stuck in there forever if you don't poke around a bit. Don't be a yolk of sadness, people. There's actually a scientifically proven way to break that membrane and the next step I'm about to reveal to you is my version: the one that worked for me.

I discovered it by accident, in a fit of rage actually. But alchemy ensued nonetheless. Rage can be useful, of course – the same as any other emotion. Just ask George Crum – the star of my favourite rage-based story. George was an African-American chef in New York state back in the late 1800s. There are a few versions of his story, but let me tell you the one I like best …

One day, a customer at George's restaurant sent his roast potatoes back to the kitchen, claiming they were too thick and soggy. Obligingly, George recut and recooked the potatoes and sent them back to the table. The customer protested they were *still* too thick and soggy. 'I do declare, these vegetables are a whole mess of dreadful!' is what I like to imagine he said.

At this point, George – irate, as you can well envisage – decided to cut those cantankerous little man's potatoes *so* thin and fry them *so* crispy, the customer would not only not be able to protest any longer, he'd have inedible potatoes to boot.

However, not only did Mr Cantankerous not complain about his overcooked potatoes, he raved about them almost non-stop from that point forward. And thus, the first commercial potato chip was born.

So even negative emotions can lead to positive ends. Ends like salt and vinegar chips. *Salt and vinegar chips, people!* Ridiculous things having disarming ends is the name of the game here. Which brings me to our first activity.

After I started chemo and my hair fell out, I was feeling a little sorry for myself. I was newly single and didn't see much chance that would be changing any time soon. However, I needed some new underwear for my upcoming hospital stays as neither the grundies with the holes in them nor the red lacy ones I had in my arsenal were going to cut it.

Put quite simply, entering a lingerie shop when you're unattached and in the eye of a cancer storm is excruciating. In every direction I looked, I saw physical reminders of what I didn't have. Not only could I only fill out half a bra, but my mind could see nothing but sexy smalls clearly destined for third dates. The displays were peppered with the occasional granny pantie too, but my single brain would only see them as 'long-term-relationship undies' and they'd mock me in much the same way.

In the end, I settled on the only thing that spoke to me that day. And I'm extremely glad I did. Because that decision led me to a place that was more positive than I could have imagined and, through some Hansel and Gretel–ing, to places that surprise me even today.

I bought superhero underwear. And I suggest you do too.

Wonder Woman, Spider-Man – whatever your flavour. If Disney princesses are more your thing, go nuts. I'd also accept Teenage Mutant Ninja Turtles or The Muppets. Even Sesame Street would be a goer. SpongeBob SquarePants understandably does quite the range too, I believe. Essentially, the more ridiculous the better.

Right now, this probably feels about as useful as a condom vending machine in the Vatican, but this is just the first crumb. And if you don't pick it up, you'll have a lot more trouble finding the second one.

Now try this: **wear superhero underwear**

So why superhero underwear?

Basically, they're disrupters. Circuit breakers. Hecklers for your pain. Psychologists call it a 'pattern interrupt' and it's a little bit of genius, in this case, in the shape of Y-fronts. I didn't know it at the time, but I'd unwittingly stumbled upon the best pattern interrupt of my life.

As a technique, it's designed to change a particular thought pattern, behaviour or situation. Behavioural psychologists use it to help modify everything from what's going on in your noggin, right down to what you do with your hands. It's a method that's long been used by advertisers and marketeers to sell you things: something unexpected is inserted into an otherwise familiar pattern. It almost always has a certain shock factor, which is exactly what gets you to pay attention to it in the first place. Like a giant billboard that says YOUR WIFE IS HOT. Then underneath it in small lettering: *Get her more energy efficient windows!* A genuine real-world example, I don't mind telling you.

But it works outside of marketing too. You know those people who do the 'year of yes'? Or those neurotic types who wear an elastic band on their wrist to snap when they have the urge to bite their nails? They're using a pattern interrupt. And from little things big things flourish.

The idea comes from a psychiatrist named Milton Erickson. You can trust his word over mine on this – he was the founding president of the American Society for Clinical Hypnosis, one of the fathers of neurolinguistic programming, and fellow to about half a dozen medical associations, just for starters.

Beginning in the 1950s, Milton started using medical hypnotherapy in his therapy sessions and he had some quite insightful things to say about the power of the unconscious mind and its ability to creatively solve our quandaries. His findings are still used to great effect today.

Most notably, he used a pattern interrupt as part of his hypnosis technique – he called it 'the handshake induction' and it involved doing something unexpected when shaking someone's hand, like pushing their arm downwards or grabbing them by the wrist instead. Because shaking hands is a formal, learned and largely subconscious behaviour, the brain and body immediately take note of the change in proceedings and are more open to other suggestions as a result. At least, that's the theory.

What does all this really have to do with my underwear? Well, whether you know it or not, you have a lot of the same thoughts, day in and day out. Most people aren't even aware of how few truly original thoughts they have. And remembering to put on underwear is up there with unoriginal thoughts. It's a very regular but forgettable occurrence. Something you likely do every single day unless you're trying to up your sperm count or get the paparazzi's attention. That also makes it the perfect time for a thought disruptor, I discovered.

Superhero underwear is silly, you see. And offensively colourful. It jolts you into happy, or at least out of self-pity, for a fraction of a second. It interrupts your pattern of pain. Reminds you to focus on what's bright and vivid with a childlike eye. It's a physical reminder of the joy you could be experiencing if you just bust out of that membrane of melancholy.

And that's how I came to use the action of pulling on my underpants to rip me out of my rut. Because that time when you step out of the shower isn't always the best of times when you're going through something physical, like recovering from surgery. There's often a moment when you catch your reflection in the mirror, naked as a streaker on the pitch, and are reminded of how much has changed. I learned very quickly that turning this otherwise quite depressing ritual into a pattern interrupt with the addition of ridiculous undies would set me up for a far more positive start to the day. Imagine for a moment, if you will, the sight of a bald woman in nothing but Yo Gabba Gabba unmentionables. It certainly takes the edge off an otherwise grim scenario.

Even now that my treatment has ended, I still use it. I apply the same disruptor to a rough day at work, a bad night's sleep or an unwelcome email. You can't take anything that seriously when you're dripping wet and looking at an upside-down picture of Big Bird.

It sounds like a Band-Aid, I know. But it's the symbol of something far more important. It's the symbol of intent. You might only have a twinge of resolve when you first find yourself in crisis, the despair is so overwhelming. But then a twinge is all you need to buy some underwear. Engage the disruptor and see for yourself.

For the record, my preference is Dr Seuss smalls. And every time I have to head in for a regular check-up – the angst of which I think perhaps only a cancer survivor can know – I'm sure to wear my lucky *Cat in the Hat* pair. They're pink and red and have a gaping big hole in the side from overuse. But those mornings, when I'm so wired from a lack of sleep thanks to my brain's insistence the cancer has returned, and I'm T minus five hours from finding out the hideous truth, I wriggle into those ridiculous pants and look at myself in the mirror. And I know that I've got this, whatever happens. Even if my malignant associate has decided to come back and sue me for running his business into the ground. Because there's still far more light in the world than there is darkness. Maybe dancing with cancer again will be my fate, but there's nothing I can do about it if it is. I just have to wear my superhero underwear, be as confident as possible, and get on with the business of getting on with it.

Your superhero underwear is just there to remind you there's happiness to be had. To be grabbed by the balls, actually. Because you can be broke, single and dying and still be happy. Trust me on this. This is something on which I do have some authority. I don't care if you're ninety-two and accustomed to cottontails, there's some superhero underwear out there for you too. Allow your genitals to be wrapped in the embodiment of amusement and observe the effect it has.

There's one other reason superhero underwear is a great disruptor ... Think about the only times in life we actually tend to buy new underwear: when it's an absolute necessity and when someone else is going to see it. I, like many women, have spent money I didn't need to spend on alluring underthings. One time I purchased a black velvet g-string it turned out I was allergic to. And did I feel good in it? I did not. I simply expected someone else would find it titillating.

Well, fuck them. Fuck anyone who isn't you. Because there are few things in your day more intimate than your underwear and it should be something you do for you and you alone. It should be a feel-good part of your routine. Superhero smalls are my little individual protest to life's many and varied curveballs.

All I can tell you is you have nothing to lose by trying this. It's alarmingly effective, it really is. And wouldn't you rather feel silly for a minute or two at the cash register in Target than be boring from the underwear out for the rest of your life? It's a universally acknowledged truth that it's always better to be fun than it is to be dull. Dull people miss out on so much of life's folly. The fact we even exist is absurd, so why not go all the way and don a pair of Jedi jocks and celebrate the fact?

As far as advice goes, superhero underwear is a good indication of what's coming for you over the next few chapters. Namely, really sweet resilience nuggets that are far less let's-sit-around-in-a-drum-circle and far more let's-get-some-vodka-and-watch-Key-&-Peele-videos. The next one involves listening to tunes. Didn't I tell you'd find these insanely easy? You can go and tidy your laundry if you think that will work for you, but otherwise – turn the page and get amongst it.

CHAPTER SEVEN

The skin of a china doll

(Or: How to find a silver
lining in anything)

All I ask for in this chapter is a couple of minutes of your time. It's the easiest request in the whole book, in fact. But do it right and you're leaps and bounds ahead of most people who are striving to be more mentally resilient. The mission, should you choose to accept it, is to get to a brain-place where your mood isn't significantly displaced by the actions of other people. And this chapter will prepare you for that like Jimmy Fallon setting up a slow jam. Getting to that point is obviously easier said than done. It's like trying to take a dump when constipated: it requires effort, concentration, solitude and occasionally some medical intervention. There is a way, though – you just need to pay extra careful attention to this next bit.

You may have already heard of something called the 'hedonic treadmill' – it's a mental model that describes the way humans seem to have a happiness set point. It predicts that no amount of weight loss or pay rises or dead relatives will change your contentment in the long run. A famous study even compared lottery winners to quadriplegics and found no marked difference in their happiness after the initial emotion of the event had died down. None!

What does that mean? In a psychological nutshell ... we're our own worst enemy.

Slightly depressing? You bet. Dreadful things, treadmills, never liked them much. So how do we get off this one? Because you do want to get off it. The benefit of which is less about maintaining a higher happiness set point and more about not letting any one incident put a dent in your emotional armour. Not the accidents or the hospitalisations, not even the gut-squeezing, soul-bruising losses. And by default, definitely not the perceived slights, like assuming the woman on the bus is staring at your double chin or thinking your waiter doesn't like you.

A lot of the research around escaping the treadmill revolves around meditation – both mindfulness and a genre called 'loving kindness meditation'. And they certainly seem to have some measure of success. But if, like me, the words 'loving kindness meditation' all in a row make you want to travel back in time to 1963 and yell at some hippies to get on with it (and get a haircut too!), then it might not be for you. There are some mini-meditations I think will work for even the most sceptical among us, though. For instance, may I present to you something I like to call ... The Montoya.

Right now, your emotions are likely being stretched across an area wider than the Amazon; your mind is trying to play a dozen different games at once. Very few of us are Bobby Fischer, however, so that's always going to be more befuddling than it is useful. Even Fischer, who many consider to be the best chess player to ever walk the earth, went mad, joined a cult and denied the Holocaust. It's just not great for your brain to be under that much pressure to perform all the time.

So quite simply, you need to start by cutting the games back to one. Like Inigo Montoya in *The Princess Bride*, the more you concentrate on a single goal, the more that goal will crystallise. Having only one primary objective means little else will be able to distract you.

If you want to have a great night out, for example, then concentrate on that. At first, it will seem like nothing could be simpler. But effective Montoya-ing means you also have to forget about someone pushing in line at the bar or your heel breaking off your shoe or even your credit card getting declined when you go to pay your tab. These things are just temporary static – you're going to have a good time anyway. You're not going to let these things detract from your main game.

Sure, Inigo was wholly bent on revenge, which isn't really the healthiest of pursuits, but he's a great poster boy for focus. Not to mention *the best character in that whole darn movie*. So make like Montoya – focus on a single thing at a time and stop wearing busy like a badge. Being able to multitask doesn't make you a more enlightened person; it just makes you a more occupied one.

Research shows that doing whatever it is that makes you pedal slower and acknowledge life with any regular frequency is one of the most effective ways we have of hopping off the treadmill. It might be yoga or prayer, a beer in silence or ten minutes in the park. Whatever it is that gives you that feeling of, 'Ohhhhh yeah. It is GOOD to be alive today.' Essentially, the device you're looking for is not getting distracted. Because distraction has been committing mass happicide in your life since you were old enough to wonder if Bert and Ernie were just flatmates. (They are, apparently – I looked into it. *Sesame Street* sent out a press release and everything.)

Our ability to simplify, focus and be calm has been decimated by being pulled by a million thoughts in a million directions. By the gait of modern life. Try thinking about the last time you were really happy ... have you got it? Okay, then what happened? You got distracted. You started wondering how long it was going to last, when you were going to be able to afford another holiday like this, what would happen if he ever left you, what if your boss didn't like your next idea, did you pay that gas bill, what's for dinner, and what were you thinking about again? And there you are, right back on the treadmill where you started. Distraction not only stops you from reaching your goal, it sucks half the fun out of any happiness you find along the way too.

But stopping yourself from getting distracted isn't a cakewalk. For instance, right now are you thinking about the hedonic treadmill or are you actually just wondering why this whole chapter is written in Comic Sans?

Comic Sans, am I right?

Okay, I'll stop now.

It probably feels like I tricked you – that I deliberately discombobulated you with typography's answer to nails on a chalkboard. But, while I may have put it in front of you, it didn't change the information I was presenting. You're the one who let yourself go off on a thought jaunt about fonts. Understandable, but probably not something Inigo Montoya would do.

The truth is distraction is something you most often do to yourself. Sure, it's easier to blame your partner, your kids, the loud neighbours, Trump, the melting polar ice caps – but it's you. You're letting yourself get interrupted. I'm not saying you need to avoid the distraction altogether; it's more that you need to learn to love the chaos and be able to block it out when it doesn't suit you. To recognise it when it's happening and embrace its disorder. That's resilience.

Just ask the guy who invented that font which distracted you so frustratingly: Vincent Connare.

Vincent has done a few impressive things in his time. He has a master's degree from the University of Reading. He designed the Ministry of Sound logo. He created font packs for both Apple and

Microsoft way back in the early '90s, which included several other well-known fonts, like Trebuchet MS and Wingdings. He's been featured in *The Wall Street Journal* and *Esquire*. But there's one thing he is most known for: being the guy that unleashed Comic Sans onto the world.

Vincent is well aware Comic Sans is the most hated font on the planet – he hasn't been living under any rocks or otherwise heavy objects. And obviously that wasn't what he had planned for his brainchild; he was just trying to create an informal typeface, for a program for Microsoft, where he was employed at the time. The font was designed for a dog named Rover, actually, who was programmed to have speech bubbles appear above his head explaining how things worked. Rover was basically the animated paperclip before the animated paperclip existed. And now you know.

As a creative guy, you can bet baby Vincent didn't dream of growing up to create a font that makes all other designers literally gag at its mere mention. But while he's now best known for something people openly loathe, he seizes that. He calls it 'the best thing he's ever done', even if it's not one of the better pieces of art he's ever produced, by his own admission.

But therein lies the secret to being positive through adversity: shrugging your shoulders when things don't go to plan, embracing the unexpected and simply making the most of the moment presented to you, whether it's shitty or not. Vincent truly isn't bothered that people abhor the thing he's most recognised for. And more importantly – as we'll soon learn – he doesn't let the fact people hate it detract from the fact people are talking about it.

He's on to something there, I think. Name another font that people have existential arguments about. Sometimes it's better to be remembered for something you believe in than to be remembered for something everyone loves. Vincent, it's fair to say, has achieved that lofty goal of not having his self-worth determined by the opinions of others.

Most of us haven't got there yet. And I don't just mean us regular folk who wear Spanx to Christmas so that our aunts don't feel the need to mention we've put on weight, sending us into a mood spiral. I also mean people who you'd think otherwise have it together. Famous people. Who do famous things. Just try asking Liam Gallagher, lead singer of Oasis, how he feels about 'Wonderwall' – the song which rocketed him to super stardom.

'I can't fucking stand that fucking song,' was his response when asked about it during an MTV interview back in 2008. Adding that he feels sick every time he hears it.

And people fucking love fucking 'Wonderwall'.

Vincent, on the other hand, speaks in interviews about how his divisive font has been used on a world cup trophy and in a Vatican photo album and had been picked up by companies including BMW and Burberry. Adding that he finds all the fuss 'mildly amusing'.

One of them certainly seems more adversely distracted than the other by things beyond their control.

So the lesson here is stop worrying about what other people say – and worse still, what you *think* other people are saying – and just concentrate on things you *can* control. Because ignoring those distractions is a sure-fire way to being more mentally resilient. It gives you a breather from the treadmill because it means you're more in charge of your frame of mind and the choices that lead to it. You're not letting other people's actions and opinions define you.

Now try this: Listen to 'Wonderwall' by Oasis

Here's my humble suggestion for this chapter: I propose you listen to 'Wonderwall' when you're done reading for the day. That glorious four-minute exemplar of mid-'90s Britpop. Depending on your age, feel free to replace 'Wonderwall' with Led Zeppelin's 'Stairway to Heaven', or Miley Cyrus's 'Party in the USA' – both are songs their artists also hate.

While you're listening to your song of choice and being overcome with feelings of youthful nostalgia, ponder the artist in question. At one time in their lives, they would have given anything for a hit song – they would have dreamt about it, yearned for it and assumed happiness approaching ecstasy would result when they got it. Then they *did* get it, and many others besides, and suddenly the very success they craved become an object of distaste.

It's not that they're ungrateful; it's just the hedonic treadmill. Remember, we're pre-wired to return to the same state of happiness no matter what happens to us. When you have a back catalogue of bangers, your new normal means you now hate the one you've heard thousands of times that overshadows everything else you do. Their happiness set point is the same – they just have new goals now.

Then start thinking about a time you wanted exactly what you have now. Perhaps you dreamt of getting married, having kids, starting your own company or living overseas. You've achieved that thing, you've triumphed – but alas, it inevitably comes with its own problems. It's all too easy to get bogged down in the minutiae of school runs or tax returns or making new friends in a strange land. That task which now seems so tedious was once part of a life which was exactly what you hoped for. You just changed your goal posts when you got it. Because you're on the treadmill too, of course. And the easiest way to quell the frustration of that is by realising you're on it. It's like an Escher painting drawn in human emotion.

The artists I mentioned are perhaps understandably a little ticked off at being defined by a song they don't consider their best work. But ask the Monica Lewinskys of the world and they'll tell you again in no uncertain terms: *you simply do not get to choose what you're defined by.* Letting go of the labels and embracing what's already happened to you in this very unidirectional thing we call life will make you a far more content person.

I suggest we all be more like Vincent: take that thing that didn't go entirely to plan and make the most of it. So maybe you did get divorced … on the day of your wedding you probably weren't expecting that would ever happen to you. If you did have an inkling at that point, mind you, it probably wasn't your smartest decision but I'm sure it was still a good party. The parting has now happened, however, so what have you learned? Perhaps you have a better idea of what you want in a partner. Maybe you've realised you don't want one at all. Perhaps it's just nice to know there's a tub of ice cream in the freezer you don't have to share. There is always, always a silver lining.

For Vincent, it's a never-ending round of speaking gigs at conferences around the world, letting everyone in on the 'best joke he ever told', even if it wasn't exactly by design. For me … well, it actually took me a really long time to figure out what cancer's silver linings were. And I had some rather profound setbacks on the way. In fact, when I first found out I was going to have to endure sixteen rounds of chemo, I sighed – rather heavily and dramatically, I have to say – and after a pause more pregnant than I'll ever be, I said, 'Well, shit … At least I'll lose those last five kilos now, right?'

You see, I was already looking for the silver lining – it just turned out it wasn't where I thought it would be.

'Um … no. You won't,' the doc replied. 'The thing about the drugs we have to give you for breast cancer is they actually make you put *on* weight. Usually around three to twenty kilos over the course of your treatment.'

I'm sorry, what? Twenty kilograms? Forty-four pounds? The weight of six newborn people?

Before I had even started, my silver lining had been ripped away from me and replaced with a pile of fat bigger than the suitcase I'd brought with me to the hospital.

In the months that followed, I looked very hard for another. Having always believed there is one in every situation, I was determined to find it. After losing my sense of taste and smell, having veins collapse on me, watching my eyebrows disappear into my soup and having toenails fall out one by one, I was really struggling for a time there. They can't actually even promise you that chemotherapy will kill your cancer, after all. It really doesn't have a lot going for it.

But then one day, many months later, when the first new hairs had started sprouting out of my head like so many tiny saplings, I finally figured it out.

For the first time in a long time, I stood back and had a good, hard look at myself, drinking in the reflection that I had spent so many months trying not to dwell on. My virgin follicles looked as though they could be blown away by a stiff breeze but screamed with potential all the same. My eyes had even begun to return to a healthy shade of white – a welcome change from the cat-pee colour I'd slowly been getting used to. Then I noticed my face. Like, really noticed it. It was completely bare; no brows, no lashes, not even the tiniest of nose hairs peeking out from my nostrils. But now that I was finally examining it carefully … there were no blemishes either. Not a pimple, not a spot, not even a freckle. No dark circles, no redness, not even one enlarged pore. Not so much as a hint I'd ever had a blackhead. In actual fact, my skin was radiant.

It turns out the same chemicals that are designed to kill those fast-growing cancer cells also kill those pesky fast-growing zit cells.

(Zit cells is not a medical term, by the way, but allow me to simplify for effect.)

In any event, I'd found a silver lining. *The skin of a china doll!* I was a living, breathing Estée Lauder commercial. Piling some makeup on top just amplified the effect. I was practically the embodiment of an Instagram filter. Probably not entirely worth enduring six months of chemo to achieve, but still, watch me glow.

Cancer was my Comic Sans: not exactly what I had planned but damned if I wasn't going to find something in there I could flaunt. And I felt so much better having found my silvery lining too. It wasn't much, but it was there.

You really, truly can find the positive in anything. And once you figure out what it is, hold on to it like Joan Rivers held onto relevancy – that woman was tenacity personified.

I will always be known to some as 'that writer who got cancer'. That will be their entire perception of me, I get that. I'd much rather be known as 'that guru who parties with Bill Murray and whom Michelle Obama calls for advice', but some things are just beyond my control. If that's what I'm to be defined by, then so be it. Accepting things that have already happened to you *and* making the most of them makes you much smarter than the average bear. Or any other large animal, humans included. So slap on your superhero undies, take it on the chin and practise Montoya-ing until you're a veritable Vincent.

Don't take too long about it, though – we're about to get into some stuff that will really blow your hair back.

CHAPTER EIGHT

The one where I do a drawing

(Or: How to figure out what motivates you)

Here's a tricky question: do you ever get the feeling your life isn't big enough? For some it starts as a niggle; for others it comes like a tsunami. But it has a way of finding you. Eventually.

For me, it started welling up in my apparently cancerous innards after my dad died. It was neither a niggle nor a tsunami – it was more like bubbling quicksand, something that felt both lethargic and cementing at the same time. It's a singularly unique event, watching someone die. For all our giant mammalian brains, we still struggle with the idea of mortality as it relates to ourselves and those we love. We know it's coming, as it does inevitably for everyone on the planet, but while that sense is akin to a fussy little rodent scratching around in the back of our minds, the reality of it is more like a catastrophic rhinoceros crashing through the centre of town.

The death of a parent is also an odd thing. Even though that's the order in which things should happen – parents going before their children – it's still disquieting. The world isn't as safe as it was before, nor as friendly. Who was I supposed to call when I got a flat tyre, found a spider or needed fifty dollars? Those were dad things. When I was thirty and forgot to pay my taxes one year, it was still my dad I called in a panic, even though I hadn't lived at home in well over a decade. Parents are like human-shaped arm floaties – losing one leaves you off kilter, flailing around in a circle.

My world felt smaller after that. Routines returned to normal but the shine had worn off somewhat. My career, my friendships – it was all a bit blah. Essentially, nothing felt big enough any more. Important enough. I suppose it's because a large dollop of joy had been forced out, like far too much toothpaste being squeezed out of a tube, an act impossible to put into reverse with any real success.

You will probably have felt this yourself at some point – that your world isn't just flat, it's concave and you're sitting right in the middle of the rut. It took me a while to work this out, but this feeling is about motivation. Your motivations have changed and you need time to reset.

On a base level, we're all essentially motivated by the same things – science tells us so. Namely shelter, sex, sleep and sustenance. All good things starting with S. Once we've got those covered, we move on – wanting safety and security. After that, skills and status. And, finally, self-actualisation.

Me? I'm clearly up to 'skills' on the ladder and working hard on my alliteration savvy. But you might be motivated by something else. Let's find out what.

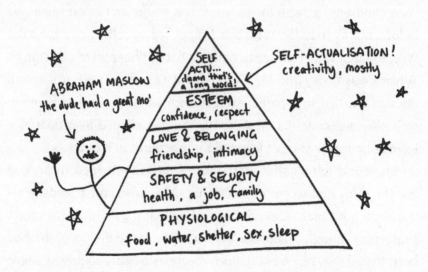

The above is a version of a diagram in every Psychology 101 textbook the world over – it's called Maslow's Hierarchy of Needs. I drew this version myself and as such I thought I'd add in some stars for effect. Makes it a little bit more *Star Trek*–y, no?

Anyway, it's based on a theory proposed by a dude named Abraham Maslow back in 1943. He expanded it many years later and other academic types have shat all over it since – mostly because it completely neglects the role social connection and collaboration play in our lives – but it remains one of the first and basic ways humans have tried to understand their own motives. And despite the fact it's not altogether factual (our countless inclinations to action are obviously far too complex to fit into a neat little pyramid), it does ultimately provides some inbuilt joy in that it's likely you have the first tier largely covered, so there's something to be thankful for right there. Food! Water! Walls! Got to be happy with that. You're already doing better than millions of other people on this planet at this point which, while depressing in its own right, is something worth appreciating. What's even more interesting, though, is you're probably self-actualising already and don't even know it.

Self-actualisation is largely about creative pursuits. Not necessarily painting or sculpting, unless that's your thing, but flexing your productive muscles in all sort of areas like your travel wardrobe, Instagram photography or dinner-party prowess. The latter might feel like you're just looking for an excuse to drink an entire bottle of wine, but it's more likely you enjoy providing for people, being the centre of a tiny community or making place cards out of doilies. You're doing something that gives you joy beyond your basic needs.

The Japanese refer to this as *ikigai* – their version of 'follow your passion' more or less, but a little more nuanced. Unlike, say, trying to turn your obsession for makeup into an income stream, your *ikigai* is somewhere at the crossroads of what you like, what you're good at and what's important to you. It's your reason for getting up in the morning. Which to me feels like a far more fulfilling pursuit than simply trying to 'do what you love' in order to fill your bank account. Japanese researchers have even discovered that finding your *ikigai* makes you live longer, so it's basically like a golden ticket wrapped in a silver lining handed to you on a diamond-encrusted platter. There's little not to love about it.

Here's a great example of someone who found their *ikigai*. There once was a woman named Heidi. She was young, pretty and as bubbly as a heart-shaped bath in the Playboy mansion. Heidi was also a beauty director for a magazine – the dream job for a large chunk of fourteen-year-olds the world over. Her day involved testing makeup, writing about makeup and being flown in helicopters to tropical islands to hear about makeup. There's no denying it was as sweet a gig as gigs get. The worst thing about her job was perhaps that she was given so much free swag she ran out of room to put it all. *The foot scrubs, the sun hats, the champagne!* What's a girl to do?

Well, one day Heidi had an epiphany. The kind you see in the movies, all lightning bolts and rays of sunshine. Heidi decided to give it all up, all the parties and celebrities and glamour, and become ... a funeral director. Yes, she wanted to swap mascara for mourners and eyelashes for eulogies. She wanted to do a deep dive on pain and introduce herself to strangers on the worst day of their lives.

Had she sniffed too much nail enamel perhaps? Gone mad with power? No, she'd just found her reason to get up in the morning. Turns out it had nothing to do with lipstick at all. She wanted to help people in a way more meaningful than recommending the best hairspray for a windy day (although, let's not mince words, that would be a good thing to know). When Heidi's life didn't feel big enough, she decided to commit herself – really commit herself – to finding her motivation until something stuck. The fact she got stuck in a funeral home is not the point. The point is her life was suddenly bigger and more purposeful than she ever imagined.

The most interesting thing about this story is Heidi isn't hypothetical at all. Heidi is actually my friend Yasemin.

'Yep! Crazy right?'

Yes, Yasemin, maybe a little.

But I get it, because while cosmetics may be some people's calling, it just didn't feel right for her. So when she found herself sitting in that rut, she actually did something about it – Yasemin Trollope up and started a small business called Rite of Passage Funerals on Australia's Gold Coast. This isn't only a tale worthy of telling because of what Yasemin gave up (did I mention the helicopters?), but because she found a way to make funerals her own. For a start, she calls them farewells. And they're bush walks and picnics and parties, and very rarely traditional in any way. And most interesting of all, she extolls the very real magic of a 'good death'. To me, this whole thing is downright fascinating. Not least of which because I'd never thought about what it would be like to be a funeral director on your first day before. Let alone one who wants to throw picnics in place of pyres.

'The most memorable moment of the whole experience was meeting my first dead person,' says Yasemin. 'It was such an initiation for me as a newly crowned funeral director to see someone who had died – I had no idea what to expect, I felt sweaty and anxious and scared. What if it was gross or I couldn't handle it? This was what I believed to be my calling, my path, but what if actually seeing a dead person turned me off it? My heart was racing when I went into the room. Inside I met an 85-year-old man who'd passed a few days before. He'd been prepared for a viewing and was propped up in bed, fully dressed and covered in a furry blanket. I stepped forward and stared. His eyes were closed and his mouth ever so slightly turned upwards, like he was smiling. I kept staring; I couldn't look away. I'd never seen anything so amazing. He looked so peaceful, so serene. There was nothing macabre or scary or gross about it. It was beautiful. He was a real gift to me. They don't all look like that, but meeting him made me realise that I was right about pursuing this after all – there is something really sacred about death. It's my "thing" – I have no doubt about it.'

On my first day in my last job I ate Turkish toast with peanut butter at my desk and wrote a script for a dog food commercial. Some of us are just better at de-rutting, I guess.

'The funny thing is this has never been motivated by money or self-importance, which feels so different from other business ideas I've had in the past,' says Yasemin. 'I was so inspired to learn, to explore, to grow ... having this idea and working on this business has motivated me in all aspects of my life. I'm a much bigger, better, wiser woman since I started on this journey. There's just no question that right now this is what I'm meant to be working on. I'm sure as time goes by and I grow, I'll be motivated by other things as well, but I know that they will all stem from this. It's only now that I've found my true calling and something that truly motivates me that I can see – and feel – the difference.'

Anyone else feeling like they should pluck their head out of the sand and take a long look around for their missing ambition? There's no denying that the feeling that you have a purpose is about the most addictive drug there is. Well, apart from those epic pain meds they give you after major surgery; those are pretty good too.

But how did Yasemin get here? How do you go from cushy job that's paying the bills to packing it all in for a crazy dream involving decaying bodies and burial wreaths?

'I just never really felt like being a beauty editor was my calling. I just fell into it – this fantasy land of fun – but I wasn't passionate about it. Because it's such a highly sought-after job, I felt extremely lucky, but looking back there was also a part of me that felt like a fraud because it wasn't a part of my identity. So I really took the time to think about what my purpose was in life; what it is I'm meant to be doing.

'One day on a hiking holiday with my family I was reading an article in *The Economist* about how crematoriums in Europe were becoming architectural works of art to try to change people's perception of death and suddenly it hit me like lightning. I started thinking about how we view death and what happens when someone dies and I realised in that moment that there was currently nothing on offer, funereally speaking, that I'd want for my family, friends or myself. I had tingles all over my body, my entire being was screaming, "Yes! This is it!" And from that moment on I've been working towards making this idea of a more modern, joyous farewell a reality.

'It was like nothing I've ever experienced before. I booked a course, spoke to as many people as I could – every day I just did something else, ticked another thing off the list. And with each step I grew more and more confident in my idea and my ability to do this work. I've always believed this is a really good idea and that just kept getting reaffirmed, which kept motivating me to move forward. In Western culture especially, death still hasn't really been confronted or embraced and I'm hoping to change that. Because from what I've found, once you really become okay with death, accept it as a reality of life and use that knowledge to motivate you to live a more rich, meaningful and purpose-filled life, then magic can happen.'

So, obviously not everyone is going to have an epiphany while reading a magazine on a mountaintop. In fact, for most of us, the initial spark is something smaller, far less grandiose. But if, like me, you've ever had someone close to you die and found yourself questioning the meaning of it all, this next part will make a lot of sense.

'Everyone copes with death differently – there's absolutely no formula at all, but what I've found is that many people do, at one stage or another, want to find more richness in their life. I've learned that slowing everything down and allowing yourself time to process your grief and what's happened can be a huge help. So often, people want to just get it over with and speed through things, but that doesn't make the feelings go away. Just slow down, sit with your pain. Finding your new normal will take time and patience, but stay with it and learn to embrace all parts of you, even the dark ones. Leaning into my trauma and emotions rather than running away from them has made a huge difference to how I live my life and how I overcome hardships. It's definitely not the easy route, but I believe it's the most effective way to move forward.

'I approach other people's trauma in a similar way in that I just allow them to feel. I don't try to fix anything or even guide them through their pain, I just hold space for them and make them feel loved, supported and safe to just feel what they need to feel in that moment. I want to empower families to take back control of the dying process. So often, in this acute phase of grief, the power is taken away from families as arrangements are made extremely quickly and their loved one is whisked away ... it doesn't need to be like that. I honestly believe that by reassessing the way we look at death, I'm going to be able to make a real difference in people's lives.'

Is it just me or is Yasemin everyone's new favourite funeral director? Move over, those guys from *Six Feet Under*. Because she's right – it's no wonder we feel so lost when we're expected to lose someone, bury them, mourn them and be back at work within the week. It's even less surprising when we go through such upheaval without the tools to deal with it properly. When you don't give yourself enough time to grieve a life you've lost – even if it's just because that person has moved out of your sphere – it's no wonder your own life doesn't feel big enough any more.

Finding your purpose in life is no easy ask, of course, and in a book dedicated to making resilience as easy as possible I'm not suggesting you go and find yourself on a month-long mountain trek or read copious back-copies of *The Economist*. In fact, I'm not going to suggest you have to find your purpose at all. I hope you do locate it somewhere on the cracked path of life, but the reality is, not all of us do. The problem is that everyone is vastly different – we might all need food and shelter but only very few of us are moved by organising wakes. Sometimes the best we can hope for is to find ambition in the everyday.

I know that's what I did.

Because while I had ample pondering time during chemo, I didn't have a lot of lofty mental power. Chemo is a lot like the worst hangover you ever had combined with the worst jet lag you ever had. As such, making any big decisions is probably ill-advised. Which is why, quite simply, I just started doing something for someone else every day. That's it. That's how I made my life feel bigger. Because while you're looking for your *ikigai* (or going through mind-dumbing medical treatment), I don't mind telling you doing something meaningfully *nice* for someone else gives you a very real sense of purpose – the impression of participating in something more important than just your own existence. There are times I think that *is* our purpose.

Now try this: **bake a pie for someone else**

Of all the little things I did – carve people's names out of fruit, send haikus, MC charity fundraisers – my favourite and most generally well-received act was baking pies. Not hard, to be honest – if you look up a recipe for blueberry pie, you'll notice it has maybe six ingredients, especially if you cheat and buy pastry. Which I suggest you do, by the way – our time on earth is short and shouldn't be spent approximating something a giant dough hook in a giant factory perfected years ago. But there's something about pies that is homey and kind and memorable. People love the shit out of pies.

I would always decorate them with words and phrases cut out of dough, topped off with real flowers and foliage, tinsel or confetti. I can remember each and every pie I've ever made. It's very meditative, making pies. Not to mention something you can do without a lot of cognitive ability or even having to change out of your pyjamas. Do use your skills, though … maybe you're not a baker but you're good at handwritten notes, have the cash to send your ten favourite people flowers or are a dab hand at mowing lawns. Research suggests doing something for someone else – 'acts of altruism', researchers prefer to call it – nudges your general wellbeing in the right direction every time.

As I made copious amounts of pies, I would ponder my future. Mull over what was meant for me in this life after cancer, should there be one. Whatever happened, I knew I'd shown pie-shaped love to all the people I really cared about. If this truly was the end, then at least I was going out in a blaze of cinnamon. Pies might have been a placeholder for more ambitious, change-the-world gestures, but they were a good one. They gave me everything I needed in the moment and allowed me to pay it forward at the same time. The smallness I felt after my dad passed away had been plugged – not by pastry, but simply by realising that *sharing* was my motive. It was the thing I wanted to prioritise in my life from this point onwards.

'Like anything in life, if you're truly committed to finding your passion and your purpose, you need to prioritise it. Even if it's just setting aside a few minutes every morning, before the craziness begins, to sit in stillness and listen to your intuition,' says Yasemin. 'It doesn't have to be anything big at first, but those small steps can add up to something. Our lives today are fuller than ever before, so it's really easy to get caught up in the noise and just roll through the days without intention. I think creating space and stillness for you to really think about what motivates you in life is key.'

Intention is the word to highlight here. If your intention for the day is just to get through it, I think you might be barking up the wrong tree, eating the wrong enchilada, peeling the wrong banana. Pick whichever idiom takes your fancy, but maybe also think about shaking things up a little while you're at it. Are you in the wrong job, wrong town, wrong relationship? No one's going to change that for you. You're going to have to teach yourself how to let go of whatever epic life-sucking entity you're holding on to, so you can move on to better things. And quickly, before you get divorced or fired or Alzheimer's. You could always have someone teach you how, I guess ... I happen to know that a little something I like to call 'chapter nine' could help you out with that, as it happens. Hint hint, nudge nudge.

And between now and then ... there's always pie.

CHAPTER NINE

Use rapscallions in a sentence

(Or: The incredible power of suggestion)

Have you ever been sky diving? Discarded a worn-out pair of jeans? Sent a child off to their first day of school? Done basically anything, ever? If so, you're already well aware how hard it is to let go. Humans are emotional bowerbirds; we instinctively hold on to most everything we feel, think, see and are told. Because we're social creatures, we're susceptible to the opinions of others. This is why we're able to band together to create great change and are capable of exponential charity. It's also why things like racism, sexism and bigotry are perpetuated, even though they make no logical sense at all.

We're complicated and it shows.

Which is why learning to let go of something you've previously believed to be true about the world isn't an easy ask. Beliefs are intangible and wide-ranging. They set up the framework you live and love by. Trying to change them is like mounting ninety-nine out of a hundred dominos, only to have to begin all over again because the set-up isn't flawless. It's so much easier to ignore the imperfections than it is to start from scratch.

I'm not talking about religious beliefs either; I'm talking about beliefs you have about society, people and yourself. Things such as 'women only like men with big bank accounts', 'a black kid is never going to grow up to be a CEO' or 'lawyers are scum'.

Shrinks sometimes call these 'limiting beliefs'. And they're real bummers, because they stop you from doing anything new that might lead to a shift in your thinking. Which of course is something you need if you want to be happier. But belief systems are created in childhood (damn you, childhood – you have so much to answer for), which means we go through life carrying these beliefs with us without question, and making decisions and seeking experiences that fit that system, rather than letting each of those experiences update our assumptions. Essentially, it's why you always choose the bad boy even though you know he's no good for you, or why you're always looked over for promotion even though you're convinced you can do the job. You justify these things in your head – he just hasn't met the right girl yet or your boss is a giant scrotum. The problem is external rather than internal. They don't call them limiting beliefs for nothing.

These mental models shape the way we see almost everything. They're what you use to help you make decisions and solve problems. As you get older and more set in your ways, you see the world through the mental model that has served you best in life. You might think this works in your favour, giving you a rosier view of the world than other people. For example, perhaps you like to think that all people are basically good. Nice thought, right? Only they're not, sadly. Some people are just cellophane-wrapped human-shaped turds. It's not great, but it's true. Thinking everyone is good and kind could unfortunately see you putting yourself in dangerous situations with rapscallions who don't have your best interests at heart. The world can be cruel in the same measure it can be magical. (Also, just quietly, how great is the word rapscallions?)

On the other hand, thinking everyone is just going to disappoint you could mean you never open up to anyone and therefore never get any sweet, sweet love in return. So that's not ideal either.

Basically: expanding your mental models is the quickest way to happiness as I see it. Short of going through a devastating life-changing event – which is actually helpful in this instance – doing this with any haste is punishing, but doable. It's one of those power-of-the-mind things. Which might sound a little drum circle-ish, but let me wow you with some science. Yes, science! Would you feel more excited about it if I put it in a cool font?

SCIENCE!

Okay, that's just Comic Sans again. Good work, Vincent.

A Finnish study published in the *New England Journal of Medicine* in 2014 detailed a trial in which a bunch of people who were waiting for knee surgery were divided in two groups: those who received actual knee surgery and those who were opened up and sewn back together, but never received surgical intervention of any kind.

I know what you're thinking – this sounds like *Grey's Anatomy* meets *Saw*, who'd sign up for this?!

Nevertheless, a bunch of knee-less wonders did and the results showed the patients who had real surgery and the patients who had fake surgery had EQUAL IMPROVEMENT. That deserves some shouty capitals.

These weren't just whingers trying to get out of footy practice either; they all had a torn meniscus and debilitating pain. I don't know what a torn meniscus is exactly, apart from sounding like a German heavy-metal band, but I'm aware it has something to do with keeping major joints functioning.

The study showed that as long as the brain *thinks* you've had surgery, it can be as good as the real thing. I'm not sure the same would be true of, say, operating on a brain tumour, but the results are pretty outlandish all the same. So if we can mimic surgery to great effect, what else can we make-believe?

A lot, is my guess.

The mind is incredibly susceptible to suggestion. Of even the tiniest variety. You know how your nose suddenly starts to itch when you pick up a large box? Your nose isn't prickling any more or less than when your hands were free; the only difference is your brain knows you can't reach it. In a split second, it realises that if it *was* itchy, you'd be in trouble and it suddenly becomes Schrödinger's snout – both itchy and not itchy simultaneously.

I'll give you another example: bald men. Put this book down and you're going to start seeing bald men everywhere. In the street, on TV, when you look over at the next car at the lights. You might even have a dream about Patrick Stewart tonight. Something *X-Men*-esque with a little Hugh Jackman on the side. Because now I've planted that little nugget in the sweet, squirrelly recesses of your brain, it won't be able to help but run with it. You might suddenly feel an urge to re-watch *Curb Your Enthusiasm* or swipe right on three hairless men in a row.

BALD MEN. It will happen to you too.

It's called the 'frequency illusion', and it's a little trick your brain plays on you in lieu of something better to do. Fancy psychological names aside, there are myriad ways the bogey man in your brain convinces you of things. But the following is my absolute favourite. It comes to you via the program manager of Harvard Medical

School's Placebo Studies, Deborah Grose. The research bigwigs at this program, hosted at Beth Israel Deaconess Medical Center in Boston, have recently discovered that even when the patient is completely aware they're getting a placebo ... *it still works.*

'We're now accumulating evidence that placebos can be administered in an open and honest manner without negating their effectiveness,' she says. 'And if deception isn't required for placebos to foster improvement, then the ethical barriers are all but removed – it opens the door to using placebos in clinical practice. There's much more to be learned about "open-label placebos", but if their promise pans out, we could see them being used in certain conditions as a first-line treatment, before embarking on a regimen that might involve health risks, side effects, and greater costs.'

So tricking your brain works as long as you want it to – this is incredibly useful information. You'll see why shortly. But I'll tell what really boils Deborah's potatoes – the work they're doing on interpersonal interaction.

'We've been operating on the belief, and there is growing evidence, that care and interaction – we call it the patient–clinician relationship – is a key component of the placebo effect,' she says. 'Most notable was a study we performed concerning people with Irritable Bowel Syndrome. There were three arms to the study: one group received interpersonal treatment that was "no-frills" – basic information-sharing with little affect. One group received an enhanced clinical interaction, including five patient-centred behaviours that clinicians were instructed to perform. And one group was placed on a waiting list and received no treatment at all. When the three groups were compared, the waitlist group improved a little, the no-frills group improved noticeably and the enhanced group improved dramatically. This demonstrated to us the amount and quality of contact with a clinician has an influence on patients' symptoms or their perceptions of their symptoms.'

Three groups, three different results. All based on the amount of actual interaction time they got to spend with the doc discussing their condition. This says to me that wanting something to work plus some human cheer squad action equals real, perceptible change.

Now, placebo studies almost always focus on medical interactions – and from my personal experience, I guarantee that a doctor who doesn't make you feel rushed is key to getting through a treatment mentally unscathed – but how does this apply outside a clinical environment? I think knowing what we do about how they work, we can use placebos on ourselves. Hear me out …

No one's immune to limiting beliefs, you see. I realised this mid-chemotherapy. We've all heard horror stories about the diarrhoea and the vomiting and the blood noses that come with this kind of treatment. When I was first told I'd need months of the most horrific intravenous drugs known to humankind, I went out and bought a gold-rimmed trash can which I planned to use as my hurl bucket. If you're going to spend the day relieving your stomach of its contents, you might as well do it with class and a gilded rim.

I expected to feel like rubbish, like hell, like I'd been cheated on by my own body which had left me for memories of a younger model. I spent several nights huddled on my bathroom floor, lolling about, feeling Prince Philip–level tired, barely able to keep my eyes open and grunting every five minutes or so for effect. I hugged my waste basket, leaching onto it for support like the face-wrapping creature from *Alien*, all limbs and desperation. I writhed, I dry heaved, I sat there on my porcelain throne awaiting the arrival of the great hoards from Colon Valley.

And nothing ever happened.

Don't get me wrong, I had plenty of toe-curling symptoms. But diarrhoea and vomiting were not part of my cancer party. Turns out all that time I spent in the bathroom would have been far better spent on the sofa finally catching up on *Game of Thrones* and coaxing my friends to bring me doughnuts. People will do that when you have cancer, it's a nice perk.

One of my limiting beliefs during this time was that I needed to be healthy to be happy. That's a pretty key one right there; you probably have it too. Most people put happy and healthy together like they're salt and pepper; you can't have one without the other. Or at the very least, having one without the other feels decidedly incomplete. But cancer taught me that belief wasn't true. Not one bit. To say that took me by surprise is an understatement.

Do you know what else you don't need to be happy? Eyelashes. Or fully functioning body parts. Or a partner. Or a father. Or money in the bank. Or a twenty-four-inch waist. Or even to have gone through life without being sexually assaulted. Just to give you some examples from my own life.

But here's what I did have: a mother who nurtured me, sisters who cared, friends who were astounding in their attentions and a medical team who were patient, adept and looked like the cast of *The Bachelorette: Let the Healing Begin.*

It didn't take me long to realise these agreeable components all had one thing in common: they were all people. All of them. Every single one. It's breathtakingly simple.

You're probably thinking, 'Well, sure – I've seen *It's a Wonderful Life* too. Obviously it's people.' But so few of us actually heed the notion that I think it bears repeating.

A healthy body would obviously be nice. As would the money or the next relationship or the bigger penis or whatever else it is you happen to yearn for. But they're such small pieces of the puzzle.

And whatever your limiting belief is – that one that's really getting in your way of having a good time – just letting it go is going to make you happier in its own right.

Now try this: **write down your limiting belief**

How did I pull myself off the floor and get out of the funk that is cancer treatment? I wrote down my limiting belief. That inhibiting brain worm that was getting in my way almost as much as the tumour.

Not in the 'I journaled my deepest darkest fears' sense, I literally just wrote it down.

You have to be healthy to be happy.

I can't tell you what your sentence will be, but you probably have some idea already. Do you secretly think you'll be happier when Prince Charming comes along? Or when you lose those last five kilos? Or when the bank finally gives you that mortgage? Write it down. And then cross it out, because it is of literally no use to you.

This process, simple as it is, uses language to change the pathways in your brain. It has a technical-sounding term for it too (because of course it does): 'neurolinguistic programming'.

Think of it like this: ever come across someone who's convinced they're too fat/ugly/awkward to be loved? These are people who told themselves something so often that they started to believe it. It works in reverse too – tell yourself you're a superstar with enough frequency and you'll start believing that. Just ask every B-grade celebrity in LA. The brain loves itself some repetition.

So here's what you do with that sentence – here's what I did – I wrote it down and crossed it out every day for a year. I skipped a few days here and there, but for the most part writing down and putting a line through a sentence that would literally take three seconds didn't seem like a giant ask. I didn't have to say it aloud or make it my mantra or put it on Twitter or even really commit to it in any other way.

It felt stupid at times. Some days I believed it. Most days the notion seemed ridiculous and I didn't. But the best part about the brain is it loves carving paths where there weren't any paths before.

Think about the footpaths the local council so diligently paved for you in your neighbourhood. I guarantee somewhere near you there's a spot where the paths intersect at a corner no one uses. Early on, someone took a shortcut. And then another someone took it and so on, and now that shortcut has worn so deep into the grass only those on roller skates or high heels wouldn't use it. A 'desire path', urban planners call it.

The brain does that too – the more a path is used, the deeper the impression becomes and the easier it is to see and use again. Repeated neural activity, a doctor would call it. Just keep thinking happy thoughts is how I would put it. When was the last time you woke up and appreciated that you were still alive? Because I do that on a regular basis. Granted I had to almost die first, but it carved a deep rut very quickly.

Figuring out what your limiting belief or mental bias is is probably the hard part. But I'm betting it almost definitely involves you beating yourself up about something. Like you're not smart enough to start your own business, or you'll never be rich, or the world is simply a cruel place to people who look like you. Figure out the one thing you really want that you don't have and ask yourself why you don't have it. That's probably your bugbear limiting belief.

And now at this point, for crying out loud, stick up for yourself. That's what the crossing out of the sentence is about. Because you do not need that negativity in your life. If someone told you your brother wasn't good-looking enough to be the face of a company, do you know what you'd say? Fuck right off with your hostility, his abilities have absolutely nothing to do with his mug. He's going to be successful at anything he puts his mind to, mark my words and hold my drink while I punch you in the junk.

You may be less or more florid, I suppose, but you would. You would say that.

So why don't you do that for yourself? Because if there's one thing I am absolutely sure of, it's that you're already equipped to be your own best cheerleader.

This is something I learned far in advance of getting cancer; I learned it from being alone, as it happens. In the ten years leading up to my diagnosis, I was largely single, from roughly my mid-twenties to my mid-thirties. And until my meeting with the Big C, this felt like the worst thing that ever happened to me. I had amazing friends, sure – but there were times I wanted to tear my hair out at the sheer length of my singledom. Why was it taking me so long to find someone I gelled with? Was it me? Was I hard to love? Am I too clingy? Not clingy enough?

And do you know what that did for me? Other than run up regular bar tabs longer than my arm? It taught me independence. In the end, after all that grief, after all those useless rhetorical questions, I finally developed a belief that I was enough. I had proven it, in fact. I'd been my own husband and lover and best friend for years, once I thought about it. By necessity perhaps, I now know full well I can go it alone without breaking down into a quivering pile. I can do anything by myself. And I absolutely will punch you in your proverbial junk if you tell me I can't. Just like a cheerleader should.

I had to do that again when I got sick. But it was a different belief, so it needed an all-new path. My placebo, it turned out, was crossing out that sentence: *You have to be healthy to be happy.*

Having science on my side helped, I suppose. As does a positive outlook, which isn't easy for everyone, I know. Some people are simply more prone to pessimism bias – the tendency, especially for those suffering from depression, to overestimate the likelihood negative things will happen to them. But even if that sounds like you, a sentence shouldn't be too much to ask. Because believing a thing really does help make it so. And not just in a spirit animal way – in a totally quantifiable, clinical way.

Here's my mate Deborah again: 'A common explanation for placebo effects concerns expectation. We anticipate feeling better and therefore we do. Another common belief is that placebos' efficacy is the result of conditioning. In other words, we've experienced relief in the past when we've received medical attention or taken medication and therefore the body has been trained to respond as before.'

Some well-worn paths at play, right there. So after you've done it once, you can do it again. As Deborah admittedly explains it, understanding how these things work in the brain involves 'tremendous complexity', but there's a lot circumstantial evidence we can use in our favour.

I knew that if I was going to die from cancer, I wasn't going to let my last months on earth be unhappy ones. What a complete waste of time that would be. Which meant that updating my belief that health was a prerequisite for happiness would have to happen with all deliberate speed. Challenging it every day by writing it down and crossing it out helped. It was a personal sugar pill I invented for myself when I had very little time and even less energy. I didn't always believe it would work or even help, but it did, because I just kept at it.

It might sound like a simplistic solution to a rather mammoth problem, but it's the rhythm of the thing that does it. It's the same principle as working out in a gym or rehearsing a tune. And it is *worth doing*. Because when you're not blessed with thinking your death is imminent, you can easily shuffle through life believing some ridiculous thing that's just getting in the way of you kicking goals. Day after day. Year after year. This isn't like putting off doing your taxes. Putting this off means making a conscious choice to stay right in the rut you're in but desperately wish you weren't. So start today. Literally, right now. Here's some space to do in, in fact.

Did you write down your sentence and then strike it out like it's two-for-one night at AMF? Good. Make that sentence submit to you like you're a dom and it forgot to give you a safe word. Because you need to work that knot out in the here and now before we get to the sexy stuff in the next chapter.

Every story needs a good romp, after all. And this one's a doozy.

CHAPTER TEN

It was Rob Lowe for me

(Or: How to change directions)

Much to my dismay – and the dismay of nerds the world over – sex in space would apparently be a complete non-event. Newton's third law (you know, the equal and opposite reaction one) means bump and grind would be reduced to more of a slip and slide. No counter thrust in zero gravity, you see. That sad fact notwithstanding, at this point in proceedings I want you to plan a trip to outer space.

Okay, so it doesn't have to be space travel *specifically*. Maybe something else equally preposterous scratches your itch. It should ideally be something as seemingly farfetched, though. What out-of-reach thing do you secretly yearn for? To be an Olympic athlete perhaps?

Ridiculous, you might say – I'm in my fifties/have one leg/weigh more than a piano and that's never going to happen.

That's not the point of this exercise – the point is to pinpoint what you'd love to do if you were in another body or had another bank account or could somehow rip Mariah Carey's vocal cords out of her glitter-encrusted neck and make them your own.

Would you have children? Write a book? Perhaps you'd like to become a surgeon. What's your one desire that's so big it feels nigh on impossible?

For my friend Cassie Workman, it was becoming a woman.

She wasn't one before that, obviously. At least not in the way most of society would deem acceptable. I first met her when she went by the name Michael and was one of the best stand-up comics I ever worked with. A storyteller of Roald Dahl proportions. I always thought of Michael as brooding and handsome and quite masculine. I had no idea Cassie was even in there.

And that, in part at least, is down to society's expectation of what sex is. What sexy is. What sexuality is. We've sectioned it all off like it's a game of Minesweeper – expect explosive opposition should you dare venture out of your carefully assigned square. Which is all quite ludicrous of us, to make it so hard to deviate. Ask anyone who's transitioned and I don't think they'd describe it as something they took lightly; a cakewalk, a lark, something they did for the attention. In fact, if I could take a stab at what the hardest thing to tackle in this life would be, I think changing sex would be way up there. Probably jostling for position with eating your best friend or killing a sibling.

For Cassie – as it is for many trans people – it was literally transition or die.

'My plan was just to keep pretending as long as I could,' she says. 'And then eventually succumb to the relentless drinking, smoking and fighting. It was a race for me, toward death. The sooner I died, the sooner I could get out. It's not that being who I am was impossible; it's that dying seemed easier.'

This is a genre of trauma many of us will never know. Then again, copious amounts of us will, in our time, know what it's like to have an open wound in our soul so big it's downright inhuman. Either way, we will all have to endure something at one point or another that seems insurmountable in its own way. Something beyond reason, without hope. Something that doesn't bear comparison. And whatever it is, that thing will be wrenching from the inside out. Dealing with the kind of trauma that feels like it's killing you softly with its very existence is obviously a deeply personal task.

'I denied it constantly,' says Cassie. 'At times more successfully than others. There were certainly times when the veneer was thinner. There were other times I was close to being honest, but I felt an enormous obligation to keep being a man. I felt like I owed my partners, and my family, and my fans this man to whom they had become accustomed. I always knew who I was, but you learn very early on that playing the role they hand you makes people happy, and I just wanted to make people happy.

'Ironically, it made everyone miserable. I was very difficult to be around, I was severely depressed, totally incapable of functioning at times, and slowly digging my own grave. I pity anyone who loved me. The process of transitioning seemed arduous, yes, but eventually it became clear to me that I couldn't give anyone what they deserved until I was honest. The people I loved the most were getting the worst of me, and I couldn't bear it. So while I knew it would be incredibly difficult – and it is – I trusted that people would be able to see a better person emerge. It *still* seems insurmountable. That's not the point, though.'

Not the point at all. Far from it. But for a lot of people, the way out of this kind of trauma feels more treacherous than trying to have a logical argument with a member of the Westboro Baptist Church.

'The first step was having a mental breakdown. Then seeing a psychologist. Then taking a year of therapy to even admit it to her.

After I came out to that first person, though, everything suddenly shifted into hyper-speed. Immediately it became imperative to catch up on as much lost time as possible. Every person I subsequently came out to made me feel exponentially better. I don't know what happened exactly, but I just didn't want to die any more. People often tell me I'm "brave", but I don't think it's brave to take the only available option to you. I didn't choose to become Cassie, really, I just stopped trying to die.'

And that, right there, is all you can do too. When something feels so indomitable you think it may swallow you whole. Stop trying to die, stop letting it kill you, just stop. Stop going forward. No other action required. At least not at first.

'Without being too "Oprah's Book Club", it's a matter of learning to love who you are,' says Cassie. 'And that's a slow process.'

Okay, let's not diss an institution this book is obviously going to be a part of. *Waves to Oprah*

'But this is absolutely the hardest thing I've ever done, and it's far from over. I went from being, as far as anyone knew, a straight white male, to being part of one of the least privileged minorities in the world, almost overnight. Although being "a straight white male" was a very traumatic experience, one advantage is that it's invisible. I do miss being able to walk down the street in relative safety without being unapologetically gawked at by idiots.

'This is incredibly hard; I wouldn't do it if I weren't absolutely certain it was what I needed to do to live. Self-care is my primary reason for doing this, and in turn I'm now able to care for those around me, but it's a complex soup of bullshit. My life is way harder than it used to be, but I'm somehow way happier and more successful. I have better outcomes in my work, I have much more satisfaction from life, I have more hope for the future. I have sort of transitioned into a more joyous and resilient version of myself.

The way forward is uncharted, so I feel I have no choice but to be optimistic. I can only compare to my life before, and the thought of going back to that is unbearable. I have optimism, and I have curiosity, for how things will progress. But what I've learned is that I'm very strong. I didn't know I was this strong, and that's comforting, because it makes the future less daunting.'

While not everyone can empathise with an existential trauma this monumental, there is so much to be learned from suffering this considered. Fundamentally: that the decision to change directions is the hardest part. To recognise that something's not working, to admit you think there's a better life – a bigger life – out there for you. Which is why I asked you what that crazy, gargantuan challenge would be for you. That thing that seems so borderline insane it could never happen. Maybe, like Cassie, it's becoming a woman. Or maybe it's something you feel has passed you by, like winning a Nobel prize or climbing Mount Everest. It doesn't matter what it is – we're not here to compare Adam's apples to oranges, we're just here to show you how it's done. Because once you figure out what it is, you take that indomitable thing and you ignore it. You don't think about what it would be like to be on that podium or on the top of that mountain or to be holding that baby. Because when you go all the way to the finish line like that, that's when it feels impossible.

What if, instead, you just took a teensy tiny step sideways – towards that ridiculous thing but a little off-centre. Something so small that nothing coming of it wouldn't feel like a failure.

For Cassie, that teensy tiny step was a pin prick.

'I went and got my ears pierced.'

A baby step with benefits.

'I was desperate to start hormone therapy, but the wait to get into the endocrinologist was more than two months, and it made me crazy. Getting your ears pierced is sort of a female rite of passage and it was important to me to make up for all the experiences I'd missed. I didn't have to change anything internally, I was already good to go.'

Obviously the difference between being male and being female is far, far more than a set of sparkly lobes. But it's a step.

For me, my existential crisis came during my lowest point in cancer treatment. Around the time my toenails started falling out. I simply hit a wall. Time felt like a soupy fog around my ankles and, quite inexplicably, the end somehow felt even further away with every hairless, lethargic week. Chemo had made my life take on some sort of *Alice in Wonderland* property. Things were more remote than they seemed, bigger than they looked and tasted all wrong. That's around the time I finally conceded my biggest fear.

You're thinking that would be dying, right?

No, the thought of dying wasn't that scary, actually. Not the actual event anyhow. Death sort of pursues cancer like a mouthy seagull, so that cogitation came with the package. I was terrified of something even more intimate than that, in a way. And it was at that point I finally entertained the deep, dark rumination I'd had since this began, but hadn't yet admitted, at least not out loud, even to myself.

I was scared I'd never fall in love again.

I could keep up the optimism when it came to slapping cancer around its ample jowls, but if I survived this round of treatment, what then? What if having both breasts amputated and your eyebrows fall out and not knowing how long you're going to live simply means no one wants you any more? I mean, that's a lot to swallow on a first date. And that's before there's even anything good to swallow.

I'd already learned that being single truly does come with a lot of perks. Even the superficial ones are a lot of fun. Like being able to eat McDonald's in bed at 3 am. And leave dirty underwear on the floor for literally weeks on end. Just to name two of my top 897 favourite fringe benefits.

But my goodness, there's a whole lot to idolise about love too. There's a reason that for every 'Single Ladies' there are three hundred thousand 'I Will Always Love You's. Fierce independence only sells so many records. And almost no long-stemmed roses. For all its lovers' quarrels and breakups and breakdowns, love has an otherworldly way of making life that little bit shinier. That little bit more purposeful. Even when we are happily single, I think we always entertain the idea of being in love again. That it could be around the corner at any moment. It's possibly the most alluring part of the human experience. Not romantic love exclusively, but loving those around us. Our family, our friends, our pets – and for a time when we're in high school, a celebrity we've never met. If you haven't crushed on someone with their own IMDb page, have you even really lived?

Coming to the uncomfortable realisation there was a very real possibility that would never happen for me again sent me into a downward spin that felt endless. I'd think I had reached the bottom only to fumble around in the dark and fall even deeper still into my despair. That impossible thing, for me, was being loved. Admired. Attractive. What if I never had another first kiss? Or romantic vacation? Or the opportunity to curl up on the couch with someone and watch TV? Millions of people take that for granted every day. But I can tell you the couch can be a very lonely place. Also a very sweaty place when you're completely hairless and it's the middle of summer, but sadly slipperiness doesn't abate loneliness.

My options for attracting potential suitors, it seemed to me, were somewhat limited. At best, I figured I'd have to wait a year –

until I was done with chemo and perhaps had some virgin lashes to bat. That gave me something to look forward to at least. Something to strive for. Being healthy and ready to fling myself onto an open market.

But I agree with Cassie on this: living like that, with your life on hold, is excruciating. I was literally just waiting for a time when I'd be fit for human consumption again.

So I took a step sideways. I downloaded Tinder.

And Bumble. And Happn. And eHarmony. You can't half-ass this kind of thing.

Where Cassie's step was a prick, mine was a click. But both were an attempt at a life that felt like a tantalising promise. Again, I don't compare our experiences, but often the way out of utter anguish is similar. It's a step at a time.

Realistically, I didn't expect much, but I so desperately needed a night out. Just one night out with someone who didn't know I had cancer. Someone who wouldn't ask me how the chemo was going or if I needed them to drop off another lasagne. I craved normalcy in whatever form I could get it. And for me – a single woman whose last companion had scarpered at the first sign of a lump – somehow nothing could be more normal than a first date. So I did just that – I fired up an app with the very robust intention of heading out for a rendezvous. It would be an experiment, I figured. A good laugh for my nurses if nothing else.

I did have a bit of a quandary, though. What pictures should I use? I didn't think my current Bruce Willis Lite vibe would garner many right swipes. But would using old photos be lying? In the end, I didn't feel I had a lot of choice in the matter, so pre-cancer me it would have to be. I'd just don my wig and pick a dark bar. Okay, a *really* dark bar.

It wasn't long before the matches came cascading in.

(Old photos, remember).

There was Sam the landscape architect, Chris the magician, Daniel the sous chef. Eventually I decided on one, a creative type. He had a kind smile, a glorious beard and syntax like a boss. I'd just go for one drink, I figured. Just one drink in order to breathe in the gloriously prosaic for an entire blissful evening. I affixed some double-sided tape to my scalp, stuck my hair-approximation on top, glued on some eyelashes and went for it. What – I reasonably thought – did I possibly have to lose?

I walked into a bar stuffed with more hipsters than a cure-your-own-smallgoods class, with some pretty severe second thoughts. How did I think I was going to fool this guy exactly? My eyebrows were drawn on entirely with pencil and, given the extreme heat of the evening, my wig could conceivably slide off at any moment. Not to mention this would be my first alcoholic drink in six months. It was like walking into an *Idol* audition with a chest infection. Or manning a kissing booth with a cold sore. I had created the perfect storm for instant and humiliating failure.

Within about ten seconds, I clocked him: my great experiment. Smart blazer, admirable posture, air of nervousness. Quite before I was prepared for it, there was eye contact. No backing out now. As I walked over to say hello, I could have sworn he looked taken aback. He's figured it out already, I thought. The non-attached hairline has given you away. An entire strip of eyelashes has fallen on your cheek. He can smell cancer.

But if he did notice something, he certainly didn't mention it. We had a drink. And another. And another. And quite a few more. Every time the door leading out to the street opened, I'd look up nervously, thinking a friend was going to stride in and bust me. 'Emma, darling – how's chemo going? Have those nipple scars healed up yet?'

We ended up on the balcony of my apartment at 3 am, sipping whiskey and making out. My one small step had turned into one giant leap for bald women everywhere.

Of course, that was also the problem. I don't know if you've ever worn a wig, but run your fingers through it and you'll pretty quickly realise something's not quite as it should be. Between trying to keep his hands away from my head, and *well* away from my fresh mastectomy, I was working overtime. I wanted him closer and further away at the same time. This had already gone far further than I had expected. But that baby step had – like baby steps do – gone down a path I had never even anticipated. Now here I was: scrambling to hide cancer meds before letting a handsome semi-stranger use the bathroom.

After eventually sending him home, I did some stock-taking. It felt like I was playing with fire. My night in the real world had been fun, but if I didn't cut it off at the knees now, it was going to run rings around me. Of course, the odds he'd even call me again were slim, I told myself, so I was probably pretty safe.

Only I was not safe. He called, I went. He called again. I went again. Three dates down and we were indulging in a long, romantic walk along the beach. And something occurred to me at that point that you might find interesting ... Men are incredibly, astonishingly unobservant. Here we were in very broad daylight and he still hadn't clocked that my brows could have been gifted to me by a three-year-old with a crayon. Ever get mad your husband didn't notice your new haircut? Don't worry – you could literally shave off your eyebrows and your nipples and he'd still be none the wiser. How the lingerie industry still makes so much money, I don't know.

But epiphany aside, this was a good and kind man. He was sweet and funny. I did not want to lie to him. I wanted to do many other things to him, but not that.

By date four, I was in a real pickle. It was then I made the decision that I wasn't going to see him again. It wasn't fair to him, I thought. What right did a cancer patient have to put someone in this position? It felt like telling him would be like asking him to hug a cactus. 'Hi, I've got breast cancer ... love me anyway?' Very prickly.

I had no right to ask that of him. But I had no right to keep it a secret either. Walking away felt like the only option that would leave everyone's dignity intact. And then the sassy little Croatian grandmother that lives in my head kicked in and slapped me. Hard. Across the face.

The opportunity for love exists everywhere, for everyone, she scolded. Why should you have less chance at love than someone with a full head of hair?

Fair point, sassy grandma ...

Is someone with mental illness less loveable, she continued? What about someone who's had a limb amputated – I suppose you think they should just be single forever?

Okay, okay.

She was right, though. I was making decisions for him. And if I didn't put myself out there I'd have a one hundred per cent chance of never seeing him again. By telling him and letting him choose for himself – well, to be fair, it was probably still a ninety-nine per cent chance of rejection, but it was far more *Notebook*-esque than just walking away.

My utter nervousness in the lead-up to date five allowed me a lot of time to think about why I was so worried. Our society still has fairly rigid ideas about what's sexy, was my conclusion. We push it out at the sides every now and again, but there's something about our pack mentality that makes it hard to make any significant headway *en masse*. Take nonchalance. I'm not sure when nonchalance became cool exactly – I'm guessing it was during the '90s because the '80s was still a very ebullient time. But eventually the Olivia Newton-Johns and Kevin Bacons were replaced with Kate Mosses and Johnny Depps and everyone suddenly seemed to be pouting and thin and disinterested. That brand of sexy is now so engrained in Western culture it almost feels like something we have to unlearn after high school. We have to retrain ourselves to be enthusiastic and responsive. To smile in photos, even.

At other times, in other cultures, all manner of equally odd things have been considered sexy. Translucent skin in Medieval Europe, for example, which saw women drawing on fake veins with blue pencil in order to look as pale and delicate as possible. Or epileptic fits in Ancient Rome, which caused acting classes to book out months in advance as people learned how to approximate a seizure. Okay, that last one I made up, but it could well be true, such is the arbitrariness of it all. At no point that I knew of, however, were bald, diseased bodies considered much of a turn-on.

'So I have something I need to tell you,' I said, almost immediately after he sat down on his bar stool at the opening of our Hail Mary date. I'd made sure I was at the designated bar thirty minutes earlier so I could get a spot near the door. It was quieter there and made for a speedy getaway when things went almost inevitably pear-shaped.

'Oh yeah, what's that?' he said.

Getting the words out was harder than eating a lightbulb for breakfast. But here's how it went down.

Me: 'I don't really know how else to say this, So, here it is … Earlier this year I was diagnosed with breast cancer.'

Him: 'Okay …'

Me: 'And I'm still in the middle of treatment … and all that involves. If you catch my meaning.'

Him: 'Okay ...'

Me: 'So, I guess I just wanted to let you know so you can, you know ... decide what that means to you.'

[Insert pause more expectant than Beyoncé at the 2017 Grammy Awards]

Him: 'Right ...'

Oh yeah. He was definitely leaving. Running for the hills. Splitting like a banana peel. And yet I kept going for some inexplicable reason.

Me: 'Right. Yep. So. You probably have a million questions?'

Him: 'Well, I guess just one actually.'

Me: 'Oh, okay, for sure. Whatever you want to know.'

Him: 'When your hair grew back, did it grow back curly? I heard that happens.'

It was at about this point that I realised he hadn't caught my meaning at all. Awkward.

Me: 'Um ... so it hasn't actually grown back yet.'

This next part still gives me goosebumps. Without his gaze floating up to my hairline (which is the first place I would have looked if someone had just essentially told me they were wearing a wig), he said ...

'Well, you know what? You can't tell. And it makes absolutely no difference to how I feel about you. I am slightly curious about your eyebrows now, though. Oh look, you're out of wine ... Another drink?'

I'd expected he'd be skittish at best, angry at worst. And that he most certainly wouldn't want to stick around to find out about my eyebrows or anything else. This was the very definition of unforeseen. He went on to ask me about how I was doing, if I needed anything and whether I'd be interested in going for Japanese food next weekend. I'd been single for years and it turned out all I needed to do to get someone to stick around was get cancer. Had I known, I'd have taken up smoking years earlier.

Just give it a week, I thought. Once we get to date seven or eight, and he starts to realise what the reality of dating someone who's going through cancer treatment is like, he'll change his ditty. Hell, he might change his mind an hour from now.

But that's okay, I decided. It's a lot to take on and I already feel like a colossal moose knuckle for even putting him in this position. Who was I to think I could date during chemo, honestly? It's like vomiting on someone's birthday cake and then still expecting them to eat it.

Oddly enough, he ate that cake and asked for seconds. There was a fifth date and an eighth and an eleventh and a sixteenth. Of course, I was still sporting a wig and gumming on my eyelashes during this time so that delivered its own delightful complications. Although My Great Experiment was now aware of my poorliness, I still tried very hard to keep his exposure to the unpleasantness at a minimum. I'd get up at 5 am and sneak into the bathroom to draw my face back on so he wouldn't have to wake up next to a naked mole rat. I'd bid him farewell at 6 am on a Monday morning, saying I had to meet a friend for breakfast, and instead get an Uber straight to chemo.

I always did get a kick out of whipping my wig off in the backseat of those rides to a pair of eyebrows shocked to the rafters in the rear-view mirror.

I wasn't trying to deceive him, just soften the blow, I suppose. I was still quite convinced it wouldn't last – and to be honest, I didn't even know if I had the wherewithal to be useful if it did – so I was just enjoying it while I felt I still could.

After date five had gone so smoothly, date six was more loaded than ... well, he was. And I obviously hadn't had sex in months by this point so, despite the eccentricities of the situation, there was no shortage of enthusiasm. None of this was what I had planned when I had said I wanted a night out all those weeks ago, and yet here we were. It was more akin to an episode of *Sex and the City* or *Seinfeld* than it was to real life. *The one where Samantha gets cancer. The one where George gets fixed up with a bald woman.*

But it wasn't the oddball spectacle that TV had told me it would be. Everything was much the same. Hands and mouths and genitals all doing what hands and mouths and genitals do. Only one thing was different, really. I'd lost all hair, everywhere, and that meant my entire body was like one big, smooth marble. I was like a dolphin fresh out of the water. I'm surprised he didn't fall off and onto the floor. They certainly never covered that in any sitcom I ever watched. And as things came to their inevitable and biblical conclusion, I lauded myself on keeping wigs and brows and respectability in place. Then I rolled over and clocked a false eyelash lodged in his chest hair like a pigeon trying to hide among peacocks. Still, a fair effort.

It was six months later when I was admitted for my last surgery – a bilateral reconstruction to put back what, in the end, two separate mastectomies had taken out. I discovered mid-chemo I had a rather lively breast cancer–causing gene, you see, and I wasn't keen on a repeat performance. The surgeons were running late that day but my new manfriend had offered to accompany me, which was actually little comfort. It was the first time I'd allowed him into the medical sanctum that was my treatment (a place where I was sans rug plus hairnet and hospital compression socks) and I was almost as nervous about him seeing me that way as I was the surgery.

When the admitting nurse asked who I wanted to put as my emergency contact, I looked over at him sheepishly and said, 'This guy? If that's okay with him? But it's also totally cool if it isn't.

We're not, like, married or anything.' I was so terrified of putting this man – this Great Experiment – in any situation I hadn't intended him to be in. Which was all of them, as it happened. But he just smiled and calmly gave the nurse his phone number.

He sat by me as we waited. An hour went by. Then two. Then three. Unfortunately, backless gowns tend to lose their novelty after about seventeen minutes. I also got more fidgety with every elongated tick of the clock. Having been through two major surgeries already, I knew what was waiting for me on the other side of those double-wide doors. A pain so full-bodied that I would struggle to breathe. An incision so wide I'd labour to move. Bruising so deep its shadow would linger months later.

Can't say I would recommend major chest surgery, if you can help it.

As My Great Experiment took it upon himself to distract me with everything in his immediate power – joking with the nurses, goading me to pose for photos and eventually even making puppets out of socks and surgical masks in an effort to make me laugh – I felt an outbreak of some kind crawl over my skin. It took me a while to figure out what it was. A hot flush was my first guess – you get those a lot when they force you into early menopause to stop your tumour from feeding on your hormones. I know – it's all shits and giggles, this cancer thing.

But no, it wasn't that.

A rash, then – an allergic reaction to the over-starched bed sheets?

It wasn't that either.

Finally, a smile crept over my face as I realised what it was. How horribly, terribly clichéd: I was in love. It had only just now dawned on me, like the solve at the end of a murder mystery party. I loved this man. I had done exactly what you're not supposed to do with the subject of an experiment and I had grown emotionally attached.

It seemed so incongruous, I recall letting out a little chuckle at the thought. This life truly is the most ridiculous, beautiful, gut-wrenching, agonising thing there is. I think as long as you experience all of those things in the right measure, you're probably doing all right. I just happened to be experiencing all of them simultaneously.

Of course, had I not just taken that first tiny step all those months ago, I never would have been here, sitting on a hospital bed staring at a man with whom I wanted to co-grow. And that step wasn't that first tryst or even really downloading the dating app in the first place – it was just deciding not to play by the rules. Not just doing what I thought I should do, what I thought people wanted me to do. Had I gone on a date that went uncommonly pear-shaped, I still think I'd be of the opinion that it was the best thing I ever did. Because I took charge of an incredibly shitty situation.

Any person who's survived the depths of something that at one time seemed unconquerable – me, Cassie, anyone who's ever had a permanent wave – will tell you that no one can make you a victim except you. And that's true.

Here's the rub, though – deciding not to be a victim certainly doesn't happen instantaneously and it rarely goes the way you expect. That's where I think most people get flummoxed. That man who comes back from a shark attack to work on marine conservation or the woman who gets raped and decides to have the child the assault left her with – they don't get to that place overnight. They have months if not years of confusing turmoil to contend with, nights spent crying themselves to sleep. These people don't become the incredibly robust human beings they are within seconds of their trauma. They work at it long, hard and with a constant inner monologue that says 'You're bigger than this'.

The decision not to suffer your circumstance isn't a lightbulb moment the way a made-for-TV movie about domestic violence makes it out to be – a peppy montage of kickboxing lessons and a swishy new ponytail and you're good to go. It's slow and aching and takes years of repeated self-convincing. Most pointedly, you have to get to a place where you genuinely don't mind if you fail. When you're not even thinking about the outcome any more. You already know it will be a win either way because you chose to look forward instead of backward.

This is a very distressing and lonely process. But the glow that decision gives you is the X-factor. An aura that has nothing to do with talent and a lot to do with an unwavering resoluteness. It's a type of evanescent bravery other people can't quite put their finger on. I don't have any forensic evidence to this effect, but I dare say that's why this relationship stuck where others fell by the wayside. Because I was there for the moment, not the destination. Because I didn't predict or even really care about our landing place. That, unfortunately for the relationship-seeking among us, is something that's hard to fake. But it's not impossible to achieve by design, not for anyone.

Now try this: plan a trip to space

Whether it's to space, Base Camp or – like me – headlong into the world of dating again, whatever your whopper of a goal, commit to it. The decision to practise complete and reckless optimism always starts with a single step up a very long ladder.

My step saw me flinging my already battered body into choppy waters at a time when most people were recommending

I lay low. Cassie's was much the same, albeit different waters on a different day. Your step will be slightly different again. But it will be small, remember that. It might be to get out of bed. Or it might be deleting a number. Perhaps it's going for a walk. It will be deceptively simple, whatever it is. But why not go for gold knowing you'll probably have to settle for silver? The glory is so often in the attempt, it honestly doesn't matter what the outcome is.

'It would be a shame to ruin your future to spite your past,' agrees Cassie. 'You have so much to learn from your challenges. Be there for them, and take notes.'

So ... who else feels like a stiff drink and a light metaphysical fumigation right about how? Good, because that's what we have coming up next. BYOBB.

Bring your own booze, badass.

CHAPTER ELEVEN

Any way you slice it
(Or: How to find balance)

There are copious blogs and books and boorish people who claim successful types all have a certain set of behaviours in common. They all get up at 5.30 am and meditate. Or they all eat dry toast and lemon water for breakfast. Or they all wear blue jeans and black shirts. Extolling these virtues implies there's some kind of fortune-telling formula for success. Which is a swell idea. How nice would it be to eat some wholewheat toast, pull on some Levis and morph into a booming start-up success story?

The kind of people they're talking about, however – the Steve Jobs and Elon Musks of the planet – are highly motivated people. They're inspired by a hunger to understand the world. A brain worm that drives them to ask and seek and build. So the trick is really figuring out what you're inspired by. Only then will you be successful enough to have people care about what you eat for breakfast.

Personally, I'm far more motivated by a trip to the Maldives than I am by running a multimillion dollar company. I'm also never getting up at 5.30 am for anything and I look ridiculous in turtlenecks. I can't squeeze myself into the success mould that works so well for the aforementioned progress pin-ups.

But does that mean I'm not successful? It does not. And emulating others isn't going to make you successful either.

I'll be square with you – figuring out what you're motivated by is no paltry project. There is literally no life hack for inspiration. I will tell you, however, it's likely you have your motivation inside out. Maybe you do get inspired by the hustle, but it's more likely you're actually motivated by the money and bragging rights it will afford you if it goes well. Or maybe you do want that job you interviewed for but only because you find the title of executive vice president psychologically rewarding. Thorny, isn't it?

When it comes to success, we tend to only see the slivers people want to show us; the product of their inspirations. We rarely see the sweat they put in to get there. Which leaves the rest of us constantly feeling like we're scrambling to catch up. Being better than the next guy, earning more money, climbing the ladder – these are all modern motivators that mean we work more than ever before.

As a civilised society, though, shouldn't we actually be striving towards working less hours, not more? Probably. But the problem isn't actually the hours we're working; it's the importance we're placing on that one chunk of our life strudel. Meanwhile, your personal life slice is over here getting all neglected and mouldy.

So how do you make sure the pastry is divided fairly? For most people, simply spending less hours at work isn't going to fly. Your inspiration – should you choose to accept it – is to spend more of your life than not doing things you enjoy, to find some people to love and who love you, and to be satisfied with the sum of those parts. Beyond that, don't idealise your inspiration too much. Because doing that is throwing off the entire balance of the layered cake that is your life.

Balance is usually thought to be a consideration of weight. A seesaw with two opposing forces teetering on each end. Of all the literature that's been written about work/life balance, most focus on ways to leave work behind. Telecommute, they say! Turn off your phone when you leave work! Learn to say no! These aren't even realistic for me and I'm a writer.

We tend to think of how we spend our life as an equation: time spent at work plus time spent at home equals your own personal parity. We constantly worry we're neglecting one over the other. Like an equal split right down the middle will create some sort of harmonic cadence. But that, right there, is just plain stressful. Our idea of balance is off balance.

'Like any profession, when you're attempting to reach the top, the main sacrifice that you make in pursuing your goal is *time*. All my time is primarily directed towards work. This said, I know if my time was directed towards other activities I'd stand very little chance of achieving what I have and what I continue to aspire to.'

This is Melissa Hamilton. She works in a career that requires a little more dedication than others. And it's by far the most influential thing in her life. But does that mean her balance is out of whack? I say no. Not least of which because her job *is* balance. In every measurable way. Because Melissa is a ballerina – a first soloist – with London's Royal Ballet.

'I feel when you choose to do something, you also give up the option of something else. Life is made up of multiple choices – each one with its own unique outcome. Cause and effect is always in play and your results are determined by the choices you make. Choosing to be a ballerina requires time and effort that I can't put into other aspects of my life – but these are the conscious and rewarding decisions I make on a daily basis.'

Melissa, unlike a lot of people dragging their heels through life, knows exactly what she's inspired by – which means her time is spent in an equilibrium most of us will never know. On paper, her seesaw is tipping heavily in one direction, but that doesn't mean she's neglecting the lighter end.

'Like most things, the achievement of each goal requires multiple facets within life to be successful – when one aspect goes out of line it throws off all the others,' she says.

And just like balancing on stage, the reward for getting it right is almost tangible.

'It feels like you're completely at one. Your body is completely centred, in "one piece". This gives a great sense of ease as your body isn't having to fight to find the balance. The secret is finding your centre – which will come with practice. It's something you won't be able to figure out from watching others; it will be unique to you.'

Melissa is talking about pirouettes of course, but she may well be talking about life. Whether you're inspired by work, family, golf, building muscle mass, reading books, living longer, volunteering or making the world's best pasta, you're driven by a desire to better yourself. And whatever it is, if you're doing it right it *will* take up a fair chunk of your time.

This is why balance isn't a symmetry or a parity. It's also why you shouldn't feel bad about skipping drinks to work on your burgeoning small business, or – conversely – ditching work emails to go to that birthday party. Your balance will be exclusive to you. What I discovered during cancer treatment – mostly because it's one of the only times in life one is given enough breathing space to work this out – is that the secret is actually in a *third* slice of strudel.

If work is one and personal life is another, the third delicious slice is that small piece you keep for yourself. This is usually the first to go when things get busy. You skip one bubble bath, then two, then before you know it you've got three kids, two mortgages and haven't had a bath in twelve years.

Making time for that third slice, though, will make the rest of the strudel so much sweeter.

Now try this: stay up past your bedtime

Finding time for that slice is no easy task. There are only so many hours in a day, but there are hacks and workarounds, even for the time poor. I personally found it in that curious little period between when I went to bed and when I fell asleep. That little hour-shaped wedge of the day most of us spend scrolling on our phones.

What did I do with that slice? Did I learn a new language? Write letters to loved ones? Journal the journey? Meditate my direction?

I'll be honest, I read Stephen King novels.

I think the key is just doing whatever it is that makes you forget what you have on tomorrow. Have that bath, masturbate, bake cookies, braid your hair, braid someone else's hair, give your dog a massage, play the piano – whatever it is you find the least bit meditative. Okay, you probably shouldn't masturbate for an hour a day, but you're picking up what I'm putting down. Also no screens allowed, so you can forget about an episode of *Black Mirror* or a stint behind the controls of your Nintendo Switch. It's surprisingly hard to spend an hour in silence without a screen to look at. But then that's the problem, isn't it?

The point here is to find the thing that forces you to concentrate on the task at hand and nothing else, because that's what puts those two other slices in perspective. For some people, this happens when they're doing something with their hands, like icing a cake or sanding a piece of furniture. For others, it's more about keeping the mind occupied. For me, trying to figure out what a giant turtle had to do with an evil clown and why a prepubescent gangbang was so imperative to the story was enough to make me forget I had a mastectomy in the morning. Probably not what King was going for, but I can't imagine he'd begrudge the result. It's quite a feat.

If an hour is pushing it for you, give me fifteen minutes. Just fifteen minutes before you go to bed. You might think it impossible – what with getting the family fed, doing some online banking and making sure everyone has clean clothes for the next morning – so here's where you might find some gains.

a) Ban yourself from TV on weeknights
Bank up all those trashy reality shows for the weekend. You might think it's your little daily indulgence, your path to relaxation, but it's quite the opposite. It's mindless screen time and I don't need to tell you that's worse for you than swapping out toothpaste for butter.

b) Be a grub
I've been doing this one my whole life – I am *so* ahead of the game. But when clean enough is good enough you will save wads of time. Don't leave dishes in the sink for days on end, but just do a very basic clean of your kitchen on a daily basis. And I mean *basic*. Sure, you wouldn't want your mother-in-law seeing it but is it good enough? There you go. Now go and buy a ukulele.

c) Skip the morning news
Instead, take that delightful dollop right after you get up in the morning – before you shower, before you have coffee – and do whatever you damn well please. If gardening makes you feel more centred than our friend Melissa mid-*Nutcracker Christmas* revival, then watering your plants in the AM will make your whole damn day run more smoothly.

While I like to read about things that go bump in the night, Melissa gets a little more physical. 'I love alternative therapy treatments such as reiki, reflexology, aromatherapy massage – that's when I feel I'm doing something for me.'

See, even her third slice helps out her first slice. She's so in sync she's practically a house full of menstrually gifted flatmates.

Don't get alone time confused with individualism, though. This isn't about working on your ego or intellectual domination. This is about taking all of that out of the picture so you can see the rest of what's going on in your life more clearly. For me, that time spent resetting myself had been severely lacking. And the focus I got from it took a lot of the sting out of everything else going on in my life. And this is particularly important when you're going through something traumatic – the brain simply can't handle agony twenty-four hours a day. Give that poor overworked organ a break.

What we're trying to do here is transcend your ego, or the self, completely, an idea most frequently aligned with Buddhism. In an age more narcissistic than a plane full of pop stars, this idea has both lost ground and is sorely needed at the same time. In fact, a recent study showed a quieter ego – one concerned less with self-promotion and more with the flourishing of themselves and others – was actually far more geared towards productivity and self-awareness. Buddhists use meditation and introspection to those ends; I'm telling you whatever helps you be more integrated in your own life will have a similar effect. We put so much effort into winning, I think sometimes we forget that to live peacefully is probably a far more self-sustaining and edifying goal.

So how do you know when your ego is quiet, exactly? Well, never fear – a band of psychologists have already worked it out.

Heidi Wayment, Jack Bauer and Kateryna Sylaska developed the Quiet Ego Scale back in 2015. In one of those big fancy lab-type studies, participants were asked to assess statements on a scale from one (strongly disagree) to five (strongly agree).

Those statements covered topics like how connected you feel with strangers, how you feel about new experiences, how easy it is for you to put yourself in someone else's shoes and whether you find yourself doing tasks on auto pilot. Which may just seem like the word jumble version of the Rorschach test, but when you get down to it, they are essentially all statements about identity. The higher you score on the test, the quieter your ego. Which, for the purposes of this study, describes a compassionate mind – one that's able to think clearly, have better insight about the self and better relationships with others.

For the record, a quiet ego is also associated with positive self-esteem, the ability to savour everyday experiences, life satisfaction, subjective wellbeing, psychological resilience and the feeling that life is meaningful. The research suggests it will also help you develop resilience in the face of the stresses and strains of everyday life.

I mean ... quiet ego: utopia, much?

Exactly *how* to shush that ego isn't something that's been proven in a lab, however. But thousands of years of Buddhism (and that one year I spent lying in bed pondering these things while sick) tell me doing something with all deliberate focus isn't exactly a bad bet. It's the third slice, the mastery of something that is for you and you alone. It's also hard to be obsessed with your own trauma when you're working so diligently on your personal growth one tomato plant/novel/batch of cookies at a time.

Finding the time to do this one thing is the only balancing you need to do. After that, plans about how you should be dividing your time just sort of fall into place.

And now you've got that in play, we can get down to the real mind-bending trickery I practise every day to get that happiness to stick like a barnacle to a ship.

BUT FIRST! THINGS YOU CAN DO TODAY: WHAT HAVE WE LEARNED?

Well, mostly that you can get a lot done in twenty-four hours. So try all these and be instantly better looking. Or at least less traumatised.

☆ Wear superhero underwear
☆ Listen to 'Wonderwall' by Oasis
☆ Bake a pie for someone else
☆ Write down your limiting belief and then cross it out
☆ Plan a trip to space
☆ Stay up past your bedtime

INSERT SUPERHERO HERE

RED-HOT HUMANITY HACKS

Next up: eight spiffy little tricks that will make you stronger, happier and more confident and will ultimately see curveballs bounce off you like hail off a hot tin roof.

TL;DR: how to be a whole person.

CHAPTER TWELVE

Oh Em Gee

(Or: How to have faith in people)

Trauma and upheaval do one thing to most people – other than make them cry like a kid who's just had a Happy Meal taken away from them – and that's question almost everything about the universe. God, fate, fairness – the whole chorizo.

We're pretty lousy at facing our own mortality until we're forced to – which means by the time we are, it comes in a confusing rush. It's like being in a room that suddenly fills with smoke and not being able to find your way out.

A lot of people turn to God in these moments, or their version of it. The idea that everything just ends is too much; we want more. And it would be remiss of me not to mention God as a pretty big piece of the trauma puzzle for a lot of people. But in this chapter, I want to talk about faith of a different kind. One I think everyone, regardless of theological proclivity, can get behind. What I'm talking about is faith in smaller, more earthly things. This, I find, is especially important if you're not religious. Because faith – in some form or another – is the basis of the human condition. If you don't believe in a divine being, you at the very least need to believe in humanity.

Call this brand of faith 'humanism' if you like – in fact, you probably should because that's what it's called. It's essentially a philosophy that relies on human ethics and social justice, rather than religious dogma and supernaturalism, as the basis for decision-making.

So what does that look like when it's at home?

'Think Buddhism; it's very similar,' says Anne Klaeysen.

Anne is the co-dean of The Humanist Institute, the Ethical Humanist Religious Life Adviser at Columbia University and the Humanist Chaplain at New York University. She also serves as a Leader of the New York Society for Ethical Culture and has doctorates and degrees up the wazoo. She's kind of a guardian of the humanist galaxy.

'One doesn't convert to us, because we don't have a creed from which that espouses,' she explains. 'We're not atheists. We're non-theists. It's a religion centred on ethics, not theology. People can believe in God, that's fine, but that's not part of our mission.'

It took me a while to get my head around this myself. So they're technically a religion – and you can be a member – but membership isn't crucial for you to identify as humanist, nor is it necessarily their goal. For me to fully grasp this, Anne basically had to redefine religion for me. Just your casual Tuesday afternoon activity.

'I think in the West, most people's notion of religion revolves around the worship of a supernatural deity in the hope of being compensated by a heavenly reward. Or if one's deeds are really heinous, a hellish one. I think that still tends to be what people think of when they hear the word "religion".

'We, however, have no such beliefs. As much as humanists love poetry and metaphor, we just cut to the chase and say, "Let's really look at who we are as a human species and what our relationship is to this environment. Isn't it wonderful that this accident – certain atoms coming together in a certain way – resulted in life? And isn't that enough to celebrate?" We don't need to attribute that to an outside force.

'Then we say, "So what's our job as human beings?" And our job is to be the best we can be, the most ethical we can be, to build ethical communities, to have good relationships, and to make sure those extend beyond our borders. To be a humanist means to be *for* something. And that's where I see that distinction. For me, it's not enough to be labelled an atheist. I don't think that's enough for most people. Because you're just kind of setting yourself up as being against something else.'

Righto, so – humanism: the thing you're for when you're not for the other things. Basically.

'The other piece of humanism, whether it's religious or secular humanism, is assuming responsibility for one's own actions,' Anne continues. 'And being responsible means that when we're connected with somebody – whether we're in a relationship, a community or we're working on a project together – we don't blame other people. We're not responsible for everything that's good or everything that's bad, we all have a part in it.'

Again: a basic faith in humanity.

And if humanism is her religion, then the New York Society for Ethical Culture is Anne's church. There are versions all over the world. While they don't gather together to pray, there is a similar sense of community. 'I do baby namings, coming-of-age ceremonies, weddings, and memorial services,' she says. 'We also offer mindfulness, meditation, yoga, things like that.'

You may or may not have heard of them before, but you will no doubt be familiar with some of the programs they've either spearheaded or advanced over the years. Things like the Innocence Project, which seeks to exonerate the wrongly convicted. Or

Planned Parenthood, an American organisation that provides reproductive healthcare. They currently have fingers in pies like stem-cell research, global warming, therapeutic cloning and facilitating health insurance for those who they feel need it most. On the surface at least, all things designed for the good of humankind as a whole.

'Ethics is always at the centre of our lives. How can we be better people? How can we relate to others better? Make the world a better place for everyone? How can we be good caretakers of the earth, the planet? We're all about social justice – so things like a living wage, not just a minimum wage, are very important to us. Humanism is the faith in human potential to be good, to do good. Sometimes that faith is more sorely tested than others.'

The way they deal with trauma, however, I find particularly refreshing.

'There's a lovely Buddhist tale that reminds me how we both see eye to eye on this,' Anne says.

That would be the Parable of the Mustard Seed: a Buddhist legend about death and grief. The story goes that a woman named Kisa had a young son who tragically died. Unable to accept his death, she goes to see Buddha, begging him to give her medicine to bring her son back to life. A request to which Buddha replies: 'Cool – just do a 180, head back to your village and bring me some mustard seeds from households that have never been touched by death. I'll then use them to make you a death-reversing potion. You dig?' That's not a verbatim quote but you get the gist. So Kisa did as Buddha asked, and her neighbours gave her plenty of mustard seeds (she was still carrying around her dead son, just FYI), but they also all assured her their households *had* been touched by death so Buddha wouldn't find them particularly useful. It's around then she realised not only that death was universal, but that Buddha had known this would happen all along. Cue Kisa facepalm. Her grief lessened, she finally buried her son.

'The reason I mention this story is because everyone – everyone – has lost someone at some point,' says Anne. 'So, yes – your particular loss and pain are unique to you. But it's not anything that isn't part of life.'

Death as a symptom of living: it's something we all have to accept, like it or not. But you're not alone in the living part.

You know how sometimes you get the feeling you're nothing special and no one cares? Well, you're half right. We're none of us extraordinary in our experience, but someone will always care if you let them. And that's why I think the ideas embraced by humanism are important. They centre around a belief in people helping people. As do most religions; I don't advocate one over another. Or any at all for that matter. I just choose humanism as an example that will hopefully make sense to believers and non-believers alike. A way in which everyone can get their head around there being something bigger than themselves without giving anything else up. Because faith in people is integral to getting through trauma. No one can do it alone and no one should try. In the end, people will be one of the most important tools to get you through.

That's why, in this chapter, your job is to have faith in people. For some, your trauma might stem from a person to begin with, which makes this particularly hard. But giving up on most of the human race because one individual cut you in half and walked away is detrimental to no one but you. In fact, if you're having trouble believing in humanity, you're probably surrounding yourself with dickheads.

Arguably, getting past that kind of trauma is possibly easier when you believe in a god with a divine plan – that way there's a reason for it, even if you don't know what it is yet. But what if you don't believe? What if you think all that's up there is a lot of light years and the only plan is the one you make for yourself?

That describes more of the population than you might think. Religious audits are finding more and more people identifying as either nones or SBNRs. That would be no religious affiliation or 'spiritual but not religious', in the assumed order. I'm somewhere in that meaty blob myself. So why exactly are so many people turning away from organised religion – particularly in a world that gets grittier by the day?

'Young people in particular are now feeling the religious institutions they grew up with are increasingly hypocritical,' suggests Anne. 'Hypocritical with regard to race relations, with regard to LGBT people, with regards to the death penalty, with any number of things. So we're finding more emphasis on the spiritual in that regard. And a lot of that also has to do with wanting to embrace science and discovery, but still maintain a religious temperament and community. So they're saying, "We don't want to have to check our brains at the door. We want to bring our whole selves through the door." And for a lot of people that means taking a closer look at theology.

'Take the creation narrative, for example – and all cultures and traditions have some kind of creation narrative – but we don't need to take that literally. Modern science really disputes the literal interpretation of that. So how can we, perhaps, be more poetic or more metaphorical about it? Maybe instead we just delight at the accident of evolution.'

Scientific proof is an interesting sticking point here, don't you think? It's called *faith* because it's not tangible and it can't be promised, delivered or bartered. It's conviction without proof. The only evidence it even exists is inside your own head. Yet it's a human construct we can't live without. It speaks to our cleverness and our creativity, and we use it all the time. We have faith people will treat us in a certain way, or that if we work hard it will pay off. We have faith that if we're our true selves someone will love us for it, or that if we tell our story someone will want to listen. There's a certain amount of hope in everything we do.

And that's why faith in people, in particular, is one of the most difficult things for a person to lose. It's not a remote control that will just make its appearance under the sofa. Getting that faith back is a laborious and painful climb up an insane incline. A mountain littered with tissues and empty wine glasses and vortexes shaped like Instagram feeds which are far too easy to slip into. Losing faith in people is one of those emotional hurts that makes itself known physically, like someone has snuck into your chest and given your heart a great big wedgie.

You've probably lost people while going through your great trauma, whatever it is. Everyone does. What you can't do is shrink away from the people who stick around. Or worse still, not let new people in. Above all, you have to have faith in people. So in order to shake off the bitterness and ready yourself to climb back up to the top of People Mountain, here's what I suggest ... you have to indulge in some small talk.

I know – small talk is the urine sample of the social world. Not an ideal way to spend a couple of minutes, but a necessary evil that gets results. Collectively detested yet constantly utilised. For most of us, engaging in small talk is a reflex, like driving a car or brushing our hair. Some avoid it more than others but it sneaks up on us at every party, in every taxi and on every phone call with a distant relative. But the trick to really getting something out of such an interaction – to mine some actual authenticity – is actually a fairly simple question.

Now try this: ask a stranger what they're reading

You'd be surprised how much of what a person is about you can find out from just one little query: 'What are you reading?'

Not everyone is always balls-deep in a book, of course, but most people will have at a minimum recently skimmed an article online. What did they think of it? What did they learn from it? Would they recommend reading it?

When I first started working in stand-up comedy, I'd spend hours waiting around to do a fifteen-minute set. I'd fill that time by talking to bartenders, patrons, other comedians. Every gig you'd get to meet someone new, an appearing-for-one-night-only friend who you'd get only a very brief chance to know. I've engaged in more than my fair share of small talk and I can tell you this question is *it*, it's the one – the skeleton key to getting past that initial veneer of disinterest, and the quickest way to make a meaningful connection I've found.

It's not an opener, mind you – you probably have to start with some light weather and traffic chat. But it's one of the best ways to turn a single-serve someone into a person you might tag in a meme one day. In the simplest sense, it's a humanistic olive branch. You're assuming everyone has something to contribute and you're inviting a conversation, an exchange. It's the swapping and sharing of ideas that makes our species great, after all. Imagine if the person who invented the wheel kept it to themselves? We'd never have made it out of the caves.

The more people you talk to and learn from, the bigger your world view will be, and the more you'll have to draw from. Because what any of us believe is just a tiny piece of a very gigantic and colourful puzzle. To be a secular humanist is to assume no person's piece is any bigger or smaller than yours.

Speaking of which, the other thing that really soaks my sponge about humanism is the way Anne uses the idea of this ever-expanding view to rethink maxims we always took as truth. Things you never even thought to question.

'We've all heard of the golden rule "Do unto others as you'd have them do unto you", right? Well, my personal attitude toward that is … no, thanks. First of all, it feels rather passive. And second, how would something that's good for me necessarily be good for the next person? I just think that's very presumptuous.

'What I say instead is we should choose to act in ways that bring out the goodness in others. And when we behave in that way, we bring out the goodness in ourselves as well. So we focus on a more dynamic, participatory relationship. It asks, "What is it you want of me? How can I be helpful to you?" And to me, that's so much better than just going ahead and doing something you assume is the right thing for someone else. It's about saying, "I'm going to have the humility to not assume I know what's best for you."

'For example, one of our members who sadly died two months ago had someone who was more religious offer to pray for her. And she said, "You know what? You keep your prayers. I'm sure you mean well, but I don't need them. I'll take your good wishes, but I find the prayer offensive." And obviously people don't mean to be offensive in this instance, but they don't actually realise they could be upsetting someone. Because they're a believer and it's what they would want someone to do for them, so they want to do it for others. This is why I say it's presumptuous. The same thing just isn't going to work for everyone.'

I hate to adopt the world's most overused social media caption here but: mind blown. If that cardinal rule doesn't make sense any more, imagine what else is ripe for amendment. As humans evolve, it stands to reason our spirituality will adapt in turn, in the same way our bodies, technology and social constructs have evolved. This might mean less bums on pews, perhaps, but that's exactly why religions need to advance too.

'We – like everyone else – are finding the congregational model is faltering a bit,' says Anne. 'People don't go to their churches and synagogues and mosques as much as they once did. We're all in the same boat with regard to that, so that's something we all need to think about. What kind of model is going to work as we continue in the twenty-first century?

'I think what's already happened is people are being more creative about community, and also about having a sense of mindfulness. So many people are now practising meditation, yoga – all of that has become more and more important. And so we need to be offering more of it, because what it does is expand the toolkit we have as human beings for living better lives. There's no longer this dualistic thing as with original sin where the soul is good and the body is evil. We're realising that body and soul are more holistic.'

And expanding your toolkit is exactly what I want to help you with, which is why I say go and find a stranger and ask them what they're reading. (Then tell them you're reading this book, obviously, otherwise we're never going to make into Oprah's Book Club.) That one little act will punch a hole in your day – stay and chat long enough and you might find that hole widens enough to let someone else in. It's such a simple question, but it says to that person, 'You matter. Your opinions matter. I care about what you have to say as a fellow human being with something to contribute in this otherwise shitty world.' That could brighten someone's day in ways you never get to witness.

Believing people are inherently important regardless of what gender they identify with, colour they are, mental illness they have or insult they hurl at you is what I would define as a faith. Lose that and your remaining time on this earth will be atrophied to no one's impairment but your own. Because faith in humanity is paramount to a competent heart. And a competent heart is paramount to resilience.

I don't care what your spiritual or religious leaning is any more than I care about how many toes you have or what your favourite food is. As long as you have a competent heart, your path will be a righteous one. In the most Teenage Mutant Ninja Turtles way possible. It will also mean you're ready for the next section ...

Spoiler alert: it involves pubes.

CHAPTER THIRTEEN

It's not like a regular canoe

(Or: Training your brain)

The following is much like personal training for your cranium. Because unless you do a few reps a day, you're never going to be able to handle anything in the least bit heavy.

Traditional brain training techniques typically cover things like improving memory, mental acuity and mindfulness, but I want to bring it all down a notch. Not usually something one wants to do with their brain, but I just think most of us need to start as small as possible. We're lazy and we know it.

Of course, we all know I'm not accredited by any scientific agency of note so this is just what works for me. Day in and day out. Through shit storms and calm seas.

To start with, think of the brain as a computer, a piece of hardware. It is, as far as anatomy goes. Like a great big MacBook in your head. Perhaps a MacBook Air, depending on how much time you spend taking selfies. The mind, therefore, if you follow the metaphor, is your operating system. With me so far?

It's no great leap, then, to think of the mind hacks in this chapter as being like software updates for your operating system. By updating your software regularly, your hardware runs more smoothly and it's less susceptible to viruses. And while computers can be attacked by phishing viruses and malware, your brain can be infiltrated by societal pathogens, like worrying about what other people think of you and feeling distressed about not looking like a Kardashian. The updates won't block these things from trying to worm their way into your brain in the first place, but they can stop them at the source.

The first hack comes at you via a story. The story of how my hair fell out, in fact.

You may be unsurprised to learn that waiting for your hair to fall out makes for a weird few days. You know it's coming – it's always somewhere around fourteen to eighteen days after your first blast of cytotoxic poison. So there you are, just sitting around, not really knowing what to do with yourself. Not wanting to go out on the off-chance they all fall out at once, like a moose dropping its antlers. Not wanting to wash it either, knowing that will only expedite the process. A fact which means the last moments you get with the hair you've had your entire life are actually kind of sad and smelly.

There's nothing that says 'cancer patient' more than losing your hair, though. It's an awful rite of passage for breast-cancer patients in particular, who have to endure some of the more intense chemicals in the chemo colouring book. It's also something a lot of patients feel rather keenly. When you've already had your rack mangled, having your hair and eyelashes taken away from you as well is like taking a dog's balls only to take his tail and claws too. Like you're stripping away everything that makes him a dog in one fell swoop.

So I sat, and I waited. My mother and one of my sisters had also come to camp out in my apartment to await the Big Fall. It was almost like waiting for a pet to die.

'Anything?' they'd ask every morning when I walked out of my bedroom.

'Nothing yet ...' I'd say.

'What about now?' they'd say.

'Nope, still nothing,' I'd reply.

Then, after more than two weeks since my first chemo and a full nine days of staying cooped up in my apartment, something I hadn't entirely anticipated happened. Something no one puts in the 'So you've been diagnosed with cancer' pamphlet. Something that is still one of my favourite experiences in my whole life.

'Guess what?' I said to my sister.

'What?' she replied, squinting at my head.

'I have news,' I said. 'Big news.'

Then I put my hand down the front of my pants and handed her a tuft of pubes.

'It's started!'

The look on a loved one's face when you gift them a handful of freshly plucked pubic hair is a singularly enjoyable intimacy. It's something I did more than once, it tickled my fancy so. Until I didn't have any pubic hair left, as it happens. It would always take someone a few seconds to compute what had just transpired, and even then they didn't really know what to do with them.

It's not something I'd suggest busting out on just anyone, but it was something that made the entire ordeal one of the more fun ones in my living memory. It took the bite out of the whole heavy, anticipatory thing. Before that, it hadn't even occurred to me my pubic hair would fall out with any particular ceremony. I was so focused on the more obvious head hairs, I'd forgotten all about them. The topside ones took two more days to succumb, but the never-gets-old short-and-curly joke kept me sustained until then and beyond.

It was about then I mused that you shouldn't just take time out to celebrate the good things in life; you should celebrate *everything*. Which brings me to the most effective brain deceptions I know.

In no particular order, my favourite positivity hacks are:

a) Observe the absurd

Give yourself credit for absolutely everything. Celebrate the big things, the small things, even the most ridiculous things. All those things you're used to taking for granted are things other people never got to do. Things like learning how to change a tyre, putting on your kid's nappies and taking out the trash. Celebrate it all.

How? A virtual pat on the back, a pause for reflection – anything that sees you practising your sense of accomplishment. I chose to glorify losing my pubes instead of seeing it as a rapidly smoothing omen of doom, but the same can be true of any of life's little experiences. Feel it, revere it and move on to the next ridiculous thing in this insane pantomime we call life.

b) Count to thirteen

We're all of us generally pretty obsessed with numbers. To the point that we let ourselves be defined by them. The amount of money in our bank accounts. The weight on a scale. The likes on a photo. All the wrong numbers. But we can't help it, because we define other people by those numbers too. How many followers do they have, what size is his waistband, how many drinks has she had?! We're besotted with counting. Since that isn't something I imagine we'll stop doing any time soon, I think we should start adding up the things that actually matter.

For example, did you know the average person laughs thirteen times a day? Or that most people have three great loves in their lifetime? Those are some pertinent numbers. Love and laughter feel like far better measuring sticks than money and social media, but in my experience very few people count their giggles.

Okay, so the number isn't scientifically set at thirteen. Some reports say four, others seventeen, others again twenty. But I like the juxtaposition and achievability of thirteen. And I suggest you start counting. Even if you have to laugh at your own jokes. For a while, when I felt particularly low, I would write the number of times I laughed that day in my diary next to the date. Humans are nothing if not competitive and I'd always try to outdo myself the next day.

c) Be your own bully

We're already pretty hard on ourselves – usually far harder than we are on anyone else. In fact, if we treated our friends the way we treated ourselves, I doubt we'd have any left.

There was a period during treatment when I found myself a little worse for wear. 'Who will want to be around me now?' I would say. 'I'm hairless and riddled with tumours!'

It was only one tumour, but still.

'Please stop talking about my best friend like that,' my best friend would say.

To which, I don't mind telling you, there is little right of reply. I would never say that to someone else going through cancer, so why would I say it to myself?

Since we're so good at beating ourselves up, we might as well beat ourselves up about the right things. This is particularly useful should you feel any shades of imposter syndrome. Because you will start scolding yourself out of fear as a matter of course. Your next move is then to scold your inner self for scolding yourself. It's meta, all right, but practise it and you'll see how well it works. You're constantly talking yourself out of being happy – so why not talk yourself into it instead?

It feels a little split-personality at first, but thinking about what your best friend would say to you should you voice those fears out loud is a pretty good place to start. Like I said, you can't stop thoughts from tumbling in, but you can give them a good hard slap.

So next time your inner monologue says, 'I'm not good enough,' let your inner bully reply with, 'Sweet baby Moses in the rushes, get over yourself – you are just as good as anyone else and what's more you have a butt that just won't quit!'

As it happens, all three of these little tricks are essentially part of one of the biggest self-help wet dreams we know – the one almost every guru from Freud to Ferris has extolled – CBT.

Basically: coping strategies.

You could fill a whole book with the theories and application of CBT – and many people have – but since I'm trying to make this easy for you, I'll skip most of it. Suffice it to say CBT (okay, cognitive behavioural therapy – I know, even the name is a little snoozy) has been successfully used to treat depression, addiction, eating disorders, substance abuse, phobias, post-traumatic stress disorder and borderline personality disorder, as well as traumas related to events such as death, divorce and cancer. So unless you're a Ted Bundy type, it should be at least slightly useful for you too.

The idea is that you change your thinking and you'll change your behaviour. This is a little simplistic, of course – and I tend to be of the opinion that you can't change your thinking as much as you can change your reaction to your own thoughts (see inner bully rant above) – but it's all part of the same psychological chicken soup.

We all indulge in some erroneous thought patterns. Those which tell us to minimise the good things and maximise the bad. Imagine you published a blog post online that garners eleven comments, for example – ten of them might be glowing, but it's the one negative one you focus on obsessively. This is an alarmingly universal reaction and levelling out that distorted thinking takes effort.

The reason I like CBT is that it acknowledges emotions are extremely difficult to change directly, but it gives you a way to keep them in check so they don't bust into your brain and draw all over the walls in permanent marker. There are a lot of psychologist-led approaches to this, including efforts like exposure therapy, but, as I may have mentioned ... I'm not a doctor. Which is why I concentrate on the one I do have some experience with: self-instruction.

Now try this: **admit you're being a douche canoe**

I find objectifying negative feelings infinitely useful. Objectify them like you're a sleazy '70s game-show host and they're bikini-clad briefcase girls. This means knowing when you're being a dickbiscuit to yourself and calling yourself out on it. Say, 'I'm being an absolute wankpuffin to myself today. That's because I'm angry. I'm angry because my last Tinder date ghosted me. Perhaps instead of nourishing this pity fest, I could be a little nicer to myself and go to the beach for a swim to cheer myself up. Because I'm actually worth far more than this melancholy field day I'm having.' Master that and what you're left with is the ability to be constantly aware of your own thoughts, like you're reading them in a Twitter feed. And just like Twitter, you can respond to the ones that you find titillating and discard the rest.

Even the Dalai Lama agrees with me – maybe not about the dickbiscuit part, but his thoughts on being able to deliberately select and focus on the positive are well documented. By only ever indulging the mental states that come from compassion and generosity, and putting your hand up to those that come from places of resentment and envy, you'll be disciplining yourself right into the corner of happiness by default.

And anyone can learn to train their thoughts. Especially if you start with superhero underwear and work your way up. You have so much more control than you think.

We do have to teach ourselves, though, because for some reason humans forget how to be happy at a very early age. My generation and every one after it have grown up faster and faster, trying to live exponentially bigger and better lives. To experience everything, to get more and better things, to do things our parents couldn't or wouldn't, to reach our potential and even further beyond that. All this vastness has left us unable to cope with something as simple as our own emotions, which is why using the coping strategies outlined both here and in CBT in general are more useful now than at any other time in human history.

But I'll let you in on the secret that everyone who has justifiably thought they were going to die knows ... we actually need to live *smaller*, not bigger.

It seems so simple when you're presented with the possibility that your time is up. Everything goes from being just out of reach behind frosted glass to being encased in a crystal-clear bubble all around you. But when you get to the end, I'll tell you what you'll want – you'll want less. Less complications, less stress, less stuff. It also becomes far easier not to be a duffel bag full of wangs when you're not climbing on other people's shoulders to get to the next rung; and far easier to just select what you need to be happy, regardless of what else is going on around you.

Using the mind to trick the mind is a bizarre experiment in artistic relativity, when you think about it. Like an arrow that points to itself. But it works, because the mind is far more powerful than the mind can comprehend. Ironic in the most insane measure, really. We don't have to know how it works. We just have to know that it does.

If bullying yourself into enjoying life is what it takes, then make it so. Life might be what happens to us, but living is how we respond. Don't make your canoe any douchier than it needs to be and your brain should react in kind. Ultimately, if you can palm off the pubes of life instead of crying over spilt follicles, you're going to be much more resilient to the next thing that comes your way.

Speaking of which, I really hope you're into Chris Pine, lacrosse and farts.

CHAPTER FOURTEEN

The flatulence factor

(Or: Getting back on your feet)

Who wants an Aston Martin? Anyone?

Me? Actually, not so much. I've always thought of my vehicle as something that just gets me from place to place without ever paying much attention to torque or trims. I could be driving a Ford or a Ferrari and I wouldn't really know the difference.

I've always admired car aficionados, though. The amount of money and time and thought they put into customising their plates and polishing their hoods far outweighs the passion I have for most things in life. I don't love it when they rev their engines outside my house on a Saturday night, but I appreciate that they've got a good, solid hobby.

It wasn't until my body screamed at me that I paid much attention to it either. I'd always treated it much the same as my car – as a vessel for getting around. I didn't care too much for changing the oil or banging out the dents. But thanks to cancer, I now have to scrutinise every bone and twitch in the whole place. And it turns out, once I gave it even the tiniest scrap of TLC, I quickly discovered how much the physical can affect the emotional.

Yes, I am aware this is something every yogi and personal trainer and Instagram fitness model already knows. Not to mention doctor, athlete and generally fit person on the planet. But I'd just truly never given it that much consideration before. I hadn't needed to, really – I was young and having fun. I spent far more time curling my hair than my biceps. But that pinch of TLC turned out to be moreish.

What do I categorise as a pinch? Walking for thirty minutes. Barely a crumb, right? I don't hesitate in telling you it feels more like a Guinness World Record–holding loaf during cancer treatment, but I take your point. It was also more exercise than I'd been doing with any regularity since the late '80s. But what a difference it made. Suddenly I was more aware of my muscles and lungs and even skin.

It's amazing how the smallest tweak can produce exponential results. Especially when you're consciously forcing your mind and body to play nice, which is actually something we rarely do. Even for the fit among us, we tend to use our minds to try to will our bodies into submission. Then our body plays tug o' war in return, not understanding why it gets a calorific overload in December only to have to give it up come January. When you think about it, it's like scolding a puppy for peeing on the rug yesterday by denying it dinner today. There are some conflicting messages there.

Actually, getting your mind and body to hum together has very little to do with fitness. But get the modulation right and the rest just sort of falls into place.

We actually know very little about how the mind–body connection works – only that it does. I'm guessing there's a submerged iceberg–sized portion we can't even comprehend yet, but then, that's what's so exciting about it.

I want to keep this as simple as possible, though. And when I say simple, I very much mean it. I'm never going to get up at 6 am to go running, or meditate in silence for days on end, or travel to India to find myself. If you feel the compunction to do these things, you're a more industrious person than me – but I'd personally prefer to spend that time drinking cocktails in the Cook Islands, watching every Chris Pine movie ever made and sleeping, respectively.

So how does your regular, procrastination-prone person fit in some self-enlightenment lite? Well, there's no one more lethargic than a chemo patient, so let me tell you what worked for me and it might just work for you too. But before that, let's take a trip to the other end of the spectrum for a tale from someone far more athletic than me.

Jim Moss is someone who had the body figured out before the mind. He represented Canada in not one but three different sports – ice hockey, field lacrosse and indoor lacrosse – winning gold, silver and bronze medals in international competition. In 2003, he was named Canada's National Lacrosse League's Defensive Player of the Year. In 2007, he was entered into a Sports Hall of Fame.

Then in 2009, his career ended when he just woke up one day paralysed. An autoimmune disease was the diagnosis. The doctor told him he would never walk again.

But Jim – he's a pretty peppy guy – hacked his own health and walked out of hospital six weeks later. Where my mind was always stronger than my body, Jim's story is the reverse. Where I had to get my body to comply, he had to get his brain to come around. So my conclusion is – if both a professional athlete and a sedentary writer can make the connection, literally anyone can.

Jim was in hospital when it started for him. In the process of relieving his bowels, of all things.

'There was a confluence of events that happened,' he says. 'I had a morning nurse and a night nurse. The morning nurse was helping me to the bathroom one day and she said, "You better get used to this, you're gonna be like this for a long time." Which is a standard approach for a lot of medical staff, to manage your expectations. When I say manage, they mean to minimise – but it's entirely demotivating. It took all the power that I might have in the situation out of it. My job, in her opinion, was to just accept it.

'Then later that day after dinner, a different nurse was helping me to get to the bathroom and she said, "Don't you worry about it, sweetheart, we'll get you back on your feet in no time." Immediately, like a bolt of lightning, I was like, that's exactly how I need to feel. I still get goosebumps when I think about it.'

It sounds like the plot of B movie, right – the rugged ex-athlete meets the kindly nurse who turned everything around. But sometimes all it takes is one person reaching out to another to boost their faith in humanity, and therefore in themselves. For that person to have hope means you have it too.

'I look back now and study even the phonetics, the grammar choices that she made. It was loaded with individual self-efficacy and group self-efficacy, with hope and optimism. We all had our part to play. So I shouldn't go back to my bed and just accept it, I should figure out how to play my part best,' says Jim.

'It also made me realise you can't control which nurse walks through the door from one day to the next or what mood they're in. So you better figure out how to insulate yourself from negative people and maybe even try to make them a little bit less pessimistic when you interact with them. It doesn't change the fact you're in a serious situation, but how can you make it light?'

Jim turned this insight into the impetus to start a gratitude journal. Which swiftly turned into something far bigger than he expected.

'I took my private journal and started to share pictures of it,' he says. 'Just on a Tumblr blog, which I had hoped would make it more meaningful. Then other people started to do it. Then more people. Then it was like, holy shit – this works. So many people started doing it we got to a point where we thought if we go a little bit further and structure this and make it easier, it could help a lot of people. That turned into a blog called *The Smile Epidemic*, where people shared pictures of themselves with expressions of gratitude, which turned into a happiness app, which led to a company coming to us and saying, "Hey, we're trying to improve customer satisfaction – do you think if our customer service reps used your gratitude app they'd be in a more positive frame of mind, and that would help us improve our customer satisfaction scores?" And I was like, I absolutely do. We had found a business model.'

Jim and his wife, Jennifer, then went on to found Plasticity Labs, a company that tries to give people the tools to make themselves happier from the ground up, based on neuroplasticity and other research paradigms. For those who've never heard of it, I'll let Jim give you his definition of neuroplasticity.

'It's the best news ever – the idea that you can teach an old dog new tricks; it's proof that if the brain is getting oxygen and glucose, it can continue to change. That change can be good or bad, but there are things that you can do to make it more likely to be positive. This isn't bullshit; this is science. It's only recently that we've had the technology to prove it. So I say, let's use it.'

And use it, Jim does. To great effect.

'We employ twenty people now. We've got four PhDs doing all sorts of crazy research and it all started with a concept that your smile has a utility, not just for you but for other people if you share it. It was like all this stored value was being wasted because we think simple things like that don't matter. I always thought of *The*

Smile Epidemic as being a bit like a change jar – I don't need to save $2000 from this pay check, but if I do save a little bit every pay then by the end of the year, next year's vacation will be paid for. *The Smile Epidemic* was like a change jar for happiness.'

A smile, of course, is a physical manifestation of happiness. A way for your body to express your mood. We have oodles of evidence that smiling is good for your health: upping dopamine, endorphins and serotonin. In short, smiling makes you feel like a better person. Jim's research says the same is true of gratitude, but in reverse – smile on the inside and the outside will play along.

When you're drowning in your own trauma, though, it can be difficult to find that internal smile; to think of anything meaningful to be thankful for. And when you get stumped on that, it can be a very difficult hole to dig yourself out of. Jim's suggestion is to start with a fart.

Yes, a fart.

'If you're having a hard time thinking of something, the advice is think smaller. Think fresh air – think, "At least this room doesn't smell like fart." Seriously, that's something to be grateful for. If you're having a hard time coming up with something, you're overthinking it.'

But you can't just do it once; you have to be thankful you're not in a stinky room every day from now on. You might want to change it up from lack of flatulence funk after a while, though. In fact, the more you change it up, the more effective it will be.

'Doing it with repetition signals to your subconscious brain that, "Well – looks like we're going to have to do this again tomorrow, so I better start paying attention to things so this guy has a list. That way when he sits down I won't have to think too hard about it, the list will just be ready." Being able to do this is a huge deal, because you only attend to about forty points of data out of the eleven million you're presented with on a moment-to-moment basis. If your subconscious starts paying a little bit more attention to things you might need to be grateful for, it has a huge impact.'

Although I thoroughly enjoy Jim's fart as a concept, I have an alternative if you like – what I started doing during treatment. As I've already suggested, I wasn't much for journalling. But I did find a way of taking a two-minute timeout to mull over what I was thankful for while also trying to train my mind–body lifeline to tighten up.

Now try this: look at the stars with your feet on the ground

Quite simply, I'd force myself to do just that: look at the stars with my feet on the ground. Like, the actual ground. Grass, dirt – nature, people. 'Grounding', it's often called. I've lived in apartments all of my adult life and, if you're anything like me, your bare feet touch the dirt far less than you think they do. The same generally goes for visiting the dentist and calling your mum. Before this, even when I was outside and running around on planet earth, I was almost always doing it with shoes on. Touching the ground with your feet is – for a lot of people – a bizarrely infrequent occurrence. And changing that is certainly not going to do you any harm. What might, though, is being a hermit who's found Gerudo Town in *The Legend of Zelda*, but hasn't seen a bird in a month. (I had to look up that Gerudo Town thing, but if you're a gamer you're catching my fly ball.)

Staring at the stars is one of those movie-scene scenarios that genuinely does make you feel small. The perspective it gives you is real and physical. It's much like staring out into the ocean from a small boat – the enormity is overwhelming.

The ground part I figured out when I had an allergic reaction to one of my chemo drugs and came out in a full-body rash, which led to me shedding an entire layer of skin like a large oafish snake. I have pictures of this – if you're writing a textbook about medical oddities, I'll send them to you. But when your feet are peeling off in playing card–sized sheets, shoes simply don't last very long. And one day, when out for my aforementioned thirty-minute walk, I couldn't take it any more. The shoes went in the bin, skin sheets and all. Walking home from the park that day, I suddenly rediscovered the restorative power of feeling fresh grass between my toes. Imagine! It's like when you walk outside and the sun shines directly on your face, only far more tactile and coming up through your feet. After that, I combined it with my star salutation and I was sold. It was so easy to be thankful for the earth, for the stars, for being there to experience them. Things developed quickly from there. It's hard to be pessimistic where you're so dwarfed by nature. It's entirely too humbling.

Jim tells me the reason this gelled for me where other things didn't is basically because I'm lazy. Which I do not disagree with one little bit.

'Essentially, we always start with gratitude because it's really quite easy to do and people want to see a quick win. "Show me this can work and then I'm ready to hear the next step," is what I get a lot. Because getting people to do difficult things is hard.

'If you're at a buffet and there's ice cream at the end of that buffet but it has a lid on it you have to open, studies show fifty per cent less ice cream gets consumed. That's how lazy we are. Speed bumps matter. So how can you find the smallest meaningful action that can be done with the most repetition to kickstart change?

'Complex plans are just totally unrealistic on this front. They sound great, they make a hell of a PowerPoint, but nobody believes they'll ever happen. So they won't even try. Gratitude almost seems too good to be true, but when you get to the neuroscience behind it, you understand how, while it may be simple, doing it with repetition creates positive and lasting change.'

I'm definitely in the fifty per cent that wouldn't bother opening the lid. Not to mention I'm down with electronic can openers and I don't own a single pair of shoes with laces. Jim's right – the whole earthly gratitude thing worked for me because it was easy. But it did work. Feet on grass became a type of Pavlovian path to happiness – my body has tricked my brain into being happy when my body does a specific thing. I'm basically the David Copperfield of cancer. Or, if you believe Jim, I'm just a person who figured out how to trigger my own optimism.

'Here's the difference – a pessimistic mindset says, "What *can't* I do right now because of what's missing in my life?" That's the default question. Whereas an optimistic mindset says, "Okay, what *can* we get done with what we have?"

'If you move from a momentary expression of gratitude to a habitual recording or consideration of gratitude, what you're actually building is a resource list. Because all those things you're grateful for, you have those already in your life. Whether it's friends, whether it's red wine, whether it's chocolate or baking, or that one person at work – those things prime an optimistic mindset; because if you've been consciously grateful for it, you can't say you don't have anything good in your life. You've made lists, and your brain loves lists because it creates all these neural connections. It will start telling you pretty quickly that you can't really be a dick today because you already know how great your life is. This one bad thing you're dealing with isn't going to make all these good things go away.'

Far better to have your brain to tell you not to be a dick than your friends and family, am I right? And if you're really lucky, you'll get to the point where you're actually *grateful* for your trauma. That might seem impossible, but you absolutely can train your brain to do it.

'If you look at post-traumatic stress, say a year after an event,' says Jim, 'a lot of people would do anything to go back in time to change the event, to avoid it. Whereas people who've experienced post-traumatic growth wouldn't go back and change it, because they feel like they've developed from that point, they've moved past it. They've taken their problems and they've built from them. Our thinking is that we should all be steering towards that in a really broad way, even before experiencing trauma. Why not start training people in advance to view challenges as just another way to learn something they couldn't have learned yesterday in the absence of this strength? It's absolute that you're going to deal with shit – whether it's cancer, it's a car accident, whatever – so how can we set ourselves up to succeed?'

I'm lucky; I could get there – to that point I was grateful for my trauma. It changed my life and I absolutely don't want to give it back. I started small, but I got there.

Of course, you might not be the staring-at-the-stars type so I'm going to give you some bonus options. Four of them, in fact. All of which – again – worked for me. Each one triggers certain physiological responses that will help that mind–body romance blossom.

Number one: go hang out with some animals
No word of a lie, spend some time in an animal shelter and you'll feel like the patron saint of puppies in no time. Heck, just spend some time petting your neighbour's cat. Animals are genuinely non-judgemental. People can't be, by default – we're wired to judge each other, to compare, to appraise. We can't help ourselves. Animals simply do not give a shit. If you're fat, thin, happy, sad, covered

in warts, a bit of a knuckle muppet, truth be told – they honestly don't care. Or even notice. We've bred them to be sentient balls of domesticity. Little parts of their brain are actually hardwired to light up when they see a human. Something I don't think would be entirely cuckoo to stamp into our own genetic code, if I'm honest. How nice would it be if your boss treated you the same way your dog did? Exactly. For my hill of beans, you can learn a lot more about being 'in the moment' from a kitten than you ever could from a YouTube video.

Number two: start greeting people generously
Not just people you know, mind you – everyone. Your waiter, your postman, most definitely your colleagues. And by 'generously', I mean both physically and emotionally. With your arms held open, palms facing up, smile on your face. Acknowledging people in a generous manner makes them feel good, which makes you feel good. I suspect it also does a lot more for your general health than kale ever could.

Number three: only eat until you're eighty per cent full
The Japanese call it '*hara hachi bu*' and it will make a world of difference. The Okinawan people do it and they pretty much live forever, but my goal for you is just to be more conscious of what your body is telling you. For a long time, mine was yelling, 'We're drowning in gravy and tumours!' and I wasn't listening. Pay more attention.

Number four: be categorically curious
Always let your body follow your mind's queries. Wondering what that flower is over there? Get up and go have a look. Pondering what that new cafe down the road is like? Go and find out. A lot of

the time, we let curiosity start and end in our head. Grab it by the balls and take it all the way.

Each one of these things will make you more resilient on a physiological level. And often that's something we have to relearn because, like most things, the kernels of resilience are more easily planted in our youth. A lot of us just seem to forget where we put them.

'In my case, I suppose sports really set me up to handle the biggest challenge I've ever had in my life,' says Jim. 'And neuroscience research shows our brains are most plastic when we're young – if we lay the right foundations, they're much easier to build on later in life. Kind of like learning a language. If you start learning more languages early in life, it's much easier to relearn them again later in life, even if they go dormant. So we think that these skills present a lot like a language; you can develop a fluency in being grateful. You default towards communicating in a certain way, and the science seems to support that. We're seeing huge performance improvements at the classroom level when we start laying down this emotional intelligence at a really early stage.'

But what do adults have that kids don't? Emotional baggage.

'Me, I had to completely break up with a previous version of myself,' says Jim. 'I didn't have a choice. As it happens, I'd taken a course at Stanford on forgiveness prior to my illness and it kept coming back to the impact losing something had on a person's belief in themselves. When something gets taken away from you, most people focus on what's gone instead of the space it opened up in their life, or what they could take from it going forward. I think it's easy to oversimplify this, but when we think there's a chance that we could get it back, that thing or person we lost, I think we linger longer. But when it becomes absolute, it's much easier to say, "Okay, this is my new reality." You go through this period of mourning – and I really do think it's mourning – whatever was lost, and I don't think we should avoid that. We talk a lot about happiness, but happiness means the ability to deal with difficult things, not avoid them, and to deal with them in a healthy way. So you should experience all the emotions. And grief and sadness have a part to play in our life.'

Jim's speaking my language. Because for all the good in the world, it is not your oyster and things will rarely – if ever – go to plan. Curveballs are always coming for you. Preparing yourself for that is half the battle. A lot of the remainder is being generous enough with yourself to give both your mind and body a break when manure does hit the rapidly spinning fan. Because just imagine for a second what that would look like. Flinging, say, a cow pat at a ceiling fan on full speed. That is not only going to be one hell of a mess, you're going to be finding bits of excrement in the drapes and carpet for months to come. A bit graphic perhaps, but no one would be surprised if you were to unearth a piece of dried poop in the rug the following Christmas, would they? Similarly, you have to give yourself enough time to scoop up all the detritus from your own proverbial shit slinging.

'It becomes about realistic expectations,' says Jim. 'For example, my dog died a little over a year ago, and it's the first time that's ever happened in my life. It rocked me. And I remember thinking, "What would be reasonable?" Of course I should be sad. I'm still going to go to work, but I'm just going to tell people that this is what I'm dealing with, so don't expect me to be myself and don't feel like you have to solve it for me. I think it's important to be okay with that as a process – saying I'm struggling is not a green light for all the solvers of the world to have to rush to your rescue. You have to be able to say, "Yeah, I'm down, but I'm okay with that."'

But wait, there's more! No steak knives, though – probably not a great gift for someone going through trauma, to be fair.

'After that, you say to someone, perhaps your best friend, "Hey, if I'm not coming around in two weeks, can you remind me? I don't need it between now and then. But if this starts to linger any longer than that ... I might need some help." But don't let them decide what the time frame is; you decide,' says Jim.

You're in charge of how long you mourn something; how long you need to let your brain be sorrowful and your body sleep in. But putting an expiration date on your pity parade is definitely a necessary part of training your brain into resilience. If Jim can mourn the loss of fluid movement and a career he trained his whole life for in six short weeks, the rest of us should be able to get over a breakup within the year. If this is something you're still struggling with, I think I know why – and it's the most human response there is. You're comparing yourself to other people.

Do I have a solution? You just know I do.

CHAPTER FIFTEEN

It's not that kind of diet

(Or: How to use comparison to your advantage)

Once you've realised the world isn't your oyster, it's easy to spread the blame around like it's peanut butter. The crunchy kind with lots of sharp bits. But your real enemy isn't your ex, your boss, the men of the world, the women of the world or even your own body. Not even if it's eating you from the inside out. Your real enemy is comparison.

It's another of those natty psychological attributes which make us so uniquely enlightened. Other species, at best, have a look around during mating season to clock whose feathers/horns/fins are bigger than theirs. We, meanwhile, like to correlate *everything* about our lives, whether we can see it or not. Whether it's even real or not.

It's called social comparison. I'm amazed some scientific type didn't go with something more cerebral like 'aggregated civil calibration', but let's be thankful for small miracles. And my go-to guy for 'I'll have what she's having' is Joshua M Smyth. He's a distinguished professor of behavioural health and medicine at

Pennsylvania State University. Day to day, he spends his time in a place called the Stress, Health and Daily Experiences lab. Or SHADE for short. His job is throwing shade where it needs to go. Which, if you're up with your fun young-people lingo, is also a phrase used to describe outwardly judging other people. Touché. But if we're all competing in a comparathon, Joshua is the line judge.

'The idea of social comparison has been around for, quite literally, thousands and thousands of years,' he says. 'And essentially, I think it boils down to the difference between an absolute judgement versus a relative judgement. So for example, how much money do I make? One way to look at that is just to say, "Do I have enough money to provide for my needs?" Another way is, "Do I make more or less than you do?" And it turns out those questions will lead to very different emotional responses.

'The philosophical traditions, the stoic tradition, and even much earlier traditions – Greek and Roman philosophers or Buddhism – talk about how when you start comparing yourself to other people, it leads to desires and responses that aren't helpful, as opposed to just focusing on what you need. And so social comparison is a theory but it's really broadened in its use and sophistication in the last fifteen years or so.'

Oh, the last fifteen years or so … hmmm, what else of note has happened in that time? Wait, I know – social media.

'The introduction of television probably had the first major impact on social comparison across the board. We suddenly got to see so much we hadn't seen before – so this idea of evaluating how I'm doing relative to some comparison, to the people I'm seeing on TV, became common. Now of course we've got that on steroids with social media. Facebook is kind of the low-hanging fruit, although Instagram is such a rich visual media, so it has a lot of potency as well. Ever heard this phrase "first-world problems"?'

I'll say I have, Josh. That was pretty much my life pre-cancer.

'Social media is ground zero for this. So I might say, "I don't have a boat and a lot of my friends have boats, and I feel very badly." That's an example of an upward comparison. I'm looking at people doing better off than I am and I want those things – the emotional response is negative. But of course social media only shows us curated experiences, so what we're comparing ourselves to becomes kind of rocky.'

As rocky as all those shorelines I'll never get to see from my imaginary boat, Josh – thanks for rubbing it in.

'Okay – but a downward comparison would be to say I just met a Syrian immigrant who has nothing, they've literally lost everything they own. They have no money, they have nothing. I'm incredibly lucky to have what I have. I feel very positive about that.'

Yep, feeling bad about the shoreline thing now.

'But boats and money is sort of an easy one. It gets a little bit trickier when it's health.'

Now you're singing my song. And your trauma will fit into this box too – because even if you're not going through something physically adverse, I'd hazard a hunch your emotional health has taken a pretty severe beating. It's just as easy to compare your tropical holiday on Instagram as it is to compare your dating life post-divorce as it is to compare your symptoms mid-cancer treatment. They're all paintings from the same awkward series.

'If I'm going to make a social comparison with my cancer diagnosis or my chronic disease diagnosis, I can look at people who are doing better, and I can look at people who are doing worse in terms of the same disease. I'm not dead, so that's a good thing – but I'm also not doing as well as others, maybe that's a bad thing. The portrayals of patients in things like pamphlets or ads is a big part of this. So when you go to a physician's office and you get a brochure for your asthma or your diabetes or your cancer medication, the people on that advertisement are almost always looking pretty good. They appear generally healthy and happy and well kept. But what if someone is not feeling or doing well? Is it actually helpful to show them someone doing better than them?'

Mad Men: they have so much to answer for.

'So we did a bunch of experiments and started to look the purpose of the comparison ... maybe it's not just up or down. There's the classic contrast comparison, but it turns out there's another way we can compare – which is the idea of identifying with the target. If I look at someone who's doing better and I say, what can I learn from that person? What skills or behaviours or responses have allowed them to do so well? And perhaps I can be motivated by that to take better care of myself or persist through treatment. So identifying upwards can be motivating, enhancing – it's a way of gathering skills or ideas. In this sense, identifying downwards might not be such a good thing any more. I might say, "Wow, I don't need to work so hard – I'm already doing so much better than those people." So it's actually more about how we compare, what we focus on, that will modulate our emotional responses.'

I guess what Joshua is saying is let those Insta-braggers be motivating, not depressing. You too can get a Fenty highlighter for cheekbones creamier than a summer soft-serve. Or a svelte rock-climbing profile picture if you quit just watching *Breaking Bad* re-runs all day. But, alas, you already know it's not that easy. Just having me tell you to find it motivating does not make it so.

'It's almost like: just don't think about your crappy life and don't be depressed, right? What's your problem? I think perhaps a useful way to think about it is our general approach to social comparison is like a habit – it's like how we eat or how we exercise. And over time, it shapes us and becomes a fairly crystallised response in the overarching pattern of how we live our lives. And with great effort, we can change it, particularly quickly and for short periods of time.'

It's like how going carb-free for a week is much easier than a year. And some diets are easier to stick to than others. You've probably already heard about how intermittent fasting – restricting your calories for a couple of days a week, but eating normally the rest of the time – can do wonders for your weight, immunity and general health. Intermittent dieting also appears to have some pretty natty psychological effects. People tend to get a little irritable after not eating for eighteen hours, sure – but studies have shown fasting also leads to feelings of increased pride and achievement.

I started intermittent fasting during chemo myself. Only not from food, from the internet. And it was *liberating*. As a completely unqualified research scientist, here's what I know: all that good diet stuff doesn't just work for bites, it work for bytes too.

Now try this: go on a social media diet

Think of it as the 5:2 diet for the internet. And let me tell you – of all the suggestions in this book, this one works the fastest. You will feel more resilient within twenty-four hours, I can almost guarantee it. Because if you think watching all those bloggers in their bikinis or your friends on expensive European holidays was tough at the best of times, try doing it confined to a hospital bed. It's genuine 4K resolution torture.

But life is far too important to spend it worrying about what's happening inside the virtual snow globe that is a free app on your phone. So eventually ... I just turned it off. Which is how I discovered a) when you go offline for two days without telling anyone people will think you're dead (especially if you have cancer). Sorry everyone. And b) how hard it is to fill a day without scrolling.

Have you tried it lately? You're obviously a book reader so you've got that going for you. But it is *tough*. At first, I just watched a lot of television. And I do mean a lot – sometimes up to eighteen hours a day. I don't feel great about admitting that, but it happened. We've devised a life in which the lack of a screen makes you feel more lonely than a baby elephant who's veered off course. I couldn't do a total detox, of course – I'm not made of titanium. But putting my phone down two days a week became my fasting goal. My reset button. I still do it to this day. Trust me when I say you need this in your life.

Also, for the record … Joshua is totally into it.

'I think that's a very clear mechanism to try to keep some perspective and to keep that social comparison from becoming automatic. And in a sense, what you're sort of promoting is the analogue to mindful eating. Don't just sit down and shove food in your face – think about what you're eating, why you're eating it, savour the experience, be thoughtful about the experience.'

Couldn't have said it better myself, Josh.

'And so you're saying do that with social media; that partial fasting. Other people could do it their way – for an hour a day, say. But to some degree limiting the dose. As long as it's being done in a thoughtful and mindful way as opposed to an automatic way, it could absolutely help.'

And help it does. It works because it turns a mindless pattern into a conscious enjoyment. Like denying yourself chocolate – it tastes better because you know you can't just have all you want. Remember when *Sesame Street* had the Cookie Monster tell kids that cookies were only a 'sometimes food'? Well, I'm happy to be the Oscar the Grouch who tells you social media needs to be a sometimes pastime. Try it for just one day and tell me you didn't realise how many actionable hours were actually in a day. Or that you didn't sleep better that night.

Confession: it probably won't be easy at first. You might discover you have real withdrawal symptoms and find yourself wondering what to do with your hands. I know I did. At one point, I even bought a crochet hook in an effort to do something practical with my jitters. I ate more. I showered two, sometimes three times a day. How much do I sound like a smoker trying to quit? Our grandchildren will be studying textbooks about internet addiction with the same wide-eyed wonderment with which we now look at pictures of the Radium Girls from the 1920s. How barbaric, they'll say.

'I would get you to be really mindful about it and do it differently every few days or few weeks, much like going on a diet or going to the gym. I think it's more about adaptively comparing yourself,' says Joshua.

As he's the expert, I suggest you do as he says.

But where all this starts to get really weird is when you realise most of us aren't just curating our social media – we're curating our whole lives.

'I'm quick to blame social media, but of course our disclosures are often curated as well. We do it automatically in daily life – you adjust how and what you present depending on your audience. Why do we do this? The reality is unfortunate: because we have situations where we get unhelpful or outright negative responses when we try to share experiences. The research suggests you're afforded some period of time when you experience something bad to talk about it, and then people seem to get tired of it.'

Sound like your friends after you were still talking about your last breakup eight months later? Oh. I've been there.

'There are also certain topics that are taboo and elicit negative responses. It depends on the recipient, but there are particular topics they may be less comfortable talking about or want to avoid; just generally stigmatised things. Perhaps if you're struggling with addiction or you've been sexually abused. It could also be a topic that runs counter to the belief structure of the listener. All of these things could immediately elicit negative responses or at least unhelpful responses. And there's been some work that suggests getting those responses can sometimes be worse than not sharing at all. But the insidious thing is that people learn that. They know that in the past when they shared about the experience of losing their child it made other people really uncomfortable, so they simply stop bringing it up.'

Interestingly, though, it isn't all bad. Curating your trauma might actually strengthen our social bonds in some cases.

'In some ways it's adaptive, because it allows the person to maintain social relationships or a particular social interaction they might have otherwise threatened. Of course, it's not adaptive in the sense they're inhibiting an emotion they want to share, and that's particularly problematic if they don't have other avenues in which to do that. It's good if we do it selectively, though – so speak to the right people at the right time, pruning some topics or some conversations. You just don't want to end up in a chronically inhibited or constrained state as that can be highly problematic – there are a host of problems associated with having to keep powerful emotional states, responses or challenges secret or inhibited.'

Essentially, it's a dance more complicated than *Swan Lake*. And no one wants to end up the Natalie Portman of the piece.

To help with this, Joshua has his own answer to my social media diet and, unlike me, he's researched this under lab conditions. He's even written a book about it. He calls it 'expressive writing'. Which is literally writing down everything you're feeling in stream of consciousness never to be read by anyone, ever.

'This came from our observations of people struggling with traumatic or deeply stressful events and this conundrum of wanting to share these experiences to make sense of them, but not always getting helpful responses in return. Our idea was to provide a very structured way for people to do this on their own. That way we could remove the threat of social evaluations, stigma, judgements, all of that stuff – and then structure the writing in a way that promotes people making sense of things, really focusing on the processing of a trauma without a set of social constraints.'

Basically, take the fear of being judged out of the picture and you'll get a much clearer path to enlightenment.

'We got around the problem by doing these really individually focused private writing sessions where you're not writing for another person to read or review – quite the opposite,' says Joshua. 'We wanted them to more honestly look at themselves and their emotional responses and to write about those, and then re-read it themselves and think about it without the imposed concerns of an audience.'

And you certainly don't have to have lab-issue pencils and paper to give this a go yourself. In fact, it would be a great way to spend that social media–free day you're now totally giving yourself this week.

Both of these exercises are simply designed to get you to stop automatically comparing yourself and censoring yourself and curating yourself. Not to stop doing them entirely, just to stop doing them *automatically*. Because that thing that separates us from the birds and the bees – that giant intellect of ours – will run off on some wild existential tangents if you let it.

'We have pretty incredible brains and those brains allow us to do a lot of really cool stuff,' says Joshua. 'We have imagination, we have foresight and active memory, we have the capacity to represent through symbolic imagery and do abstract reasoning – all of that great stuff. But what it also means is we don't solely exist in a stimulus response state like simple organisms do. With something like a paramecium, a single-celled organism, they're hardwired to respond when the environment produces a stimulus. With a withdrawal reflex or ingestion or mitosis or whatever. But we've evolved beyond that; we're not merely responding to our environment any more. We're responding to symbolic representations of our environment. We're responding to our *responses* to the environment. That sounds a little bit postmodern, but we're layering things onto the actual environment.'

It's like Will Smith just dropped another one of those rambling Facebook videos ... I had to get Joshua to unpack this one for me.

'Okay, so imagine I say to you, "Picture some horrible thing."'

'Like a cow-sized spider?' I say.

'Um. Sure ...'

Awkward pause.

'Your body will respond to that image, though – you'll show a physiological stress response just as vividly as if you experienced it. Our biology is therefore not only influenced by environmental stimuli – which could be anything from breaking a bone, taking a drug, having some perceived threat in our environment – but also to all of the mental imagery we replay.'

I actually dreamt about bovine-shaped spiders that night so I can attest to that. But it gets way freakier.

'Even more importantly, that mental imagery can go backwards in time. We think a lot about bad things that have happened in our past. Then we follow those images through to the future – we worry and anticipate other bad things might happen going forward. And we bear the biological burden of not just reality, but all of this created reality. So in terms of health, all of this could essentially amount to a chronic stress response, which could depress or impair normal physiological functioning; a sort of low-grade immunosuppressant.'

Could our brains be any more annoying? Unless your inner monologue speaks to you in an affected Gilbert Gottfried accent, I'd say not. And this is exactly why we need to spend all this time talking about comparison – because you're not just comparing yourself to other people, you're comparing yourself to yesterday's version of you and several future versions of you. This could not be more exhausting or unhelpful if it was all covered in already-popped bubble wrap.

'You want to be more aware of when you're doing this,' says Joshua. 'Because then you start saying, "Today is not as good as my best day ever, and it's definitely not as good as all these incredible lives I see on Facebook and Instagram, so ergo every day is shit."'

But while everything we've talked about so far involves very individual behaviour changes – put down your phone, pick up a pen – you're not going to be able to do any of it without a little help from your friends, as it were.

'Early on, a lot of this work focused on the idea that we do all of that processing by ourselves – that's it's a completely inter-psychic process. It's really only in the last few decades people have started thinking about social support and the protective nature of positive relationships and social networks. We need to talk to other people in a way that helps us understand and process emotional experiences.'

Essentially, people literally can't survive without other people. We wither at a surprisingly swift rate, like flowers without water. Prisoners in solitary confinement, for example, experience anxiety, panic attacks and disordered thinking within weeks. They pace, they're confused, they can't sleep. Suicide rates are staggeringly high. And yet a lot of us voluntarily put ourselves into a type of confinement on a daily basis. Convinced we're more connected to people than ever while actually keeping them at arm's reach – quite literally as we hold our phones in our mitts, forever rewarded by lights and vibrations, being able to text and tweet and comment on the hour, every hour, but not see a soul for days. That's our lax, Pavlovian reality. It's every dystopian future novel that ever was wrapped into one, with an extra gig of data for just ten dollars a month. So I say again, put the phone down. Your trauma certainly won't be abetted by yet another picture of a pool in LA. But take that predisposition for upwards-inflecting comparison and use it to your advantage.

'Absolutely, compare affirmatively upwards,' agrees Joshua. 'Say, no – I don't have everything in my life done yet. But I'm a little better today than I was last week. I've made some progress. I'm working towards my goals and I'm feeling better about it. And go out there and have wonderful relationships – with friends, family, find a great therapist or hairdresser or bartender who listens supportively and non-judgementally. One of the most effective ways we process trauma is by involving other people.'

Consequently: going on a social media diet, trying some expressive writing and learning to use social comparison to your advantage will not only help you climb out of whatever hole you're in, it might even help score you a free G&T when your kindly bartender empathises with your shitty situation. I think there's a little something in that for everyone, don't you?

However, one of the hardest environments in which to quell the comparathon is the one where we have to spend most of our time, whether we like it or not ... at work. That's coming up next, after a message from our sponsors.

Just kidding, I don't have any sponsors.

CHAPTER SIXTEEN

There's no place like home

(Or: How to know when to quit)

Many of us will spend one third of our lives at work. Which means an entire third of your life spent staring at screens, answering emails, going to meetings. Around 90,000 hours over your lifetime. That is, if you're lucky not to be confined to a hospital bed for years on end or stuck in jail thanks to a particularly erroneous decision. Just heaping some perspective on you like a sixteen-year-old boy unloading into a sports sock – I think sometimes we need the reminder.

But because we spend so much time earning a crust, we've become obsessed with the idea of loving what we do. We talk about it, we crave it, we pay to go to seminars about it. This is a good problem to have; it means we've reached a point in society where things are humming along nicely, actually. At least in terms of us having our basic needs taken care of. It means we can turn our gaze to other things like creativity and travel and Chris Hemsworth. And being really, truly satisfied by our work.

As such, motivational quotes have become the cryptocurrency of self-help, their popularity constantly on the rise, each of us theoretically on board even though we don't really know what it means or how it works. I tend to think motivational memes will be a social curio we will one day look back on the way we now ponder the smoking ads of the '50s and '60s. They're so of their moment, but so nonsensical at the same time. You know the kind I'm talking about – *Love what you do and you won't work a day in your life* or *Don't settle until your passion is your paycheque.* That type of thing. They're almost always written coquettishly in millennium pink type.

Well, I call bullshit on that. You do not have to love what you do for a living.

I understand why the idea has caught on like an STI at a high-school mixer, mind you – we've all come down with a terrible case of not being Beyoncé and Jay-Z, and we're collectively and awfully upset about it. We want more. We want status, we want accolades. We want to be on the cover of *Entrepreneurs Who Are Better Than You* magazine. Not a real publication, shockingly, yet we're all haunted by this idea we're wasting our lives in some way.

But we can't all love our work. It's just not realistic. For instance, do you imagine every assembly worker on earth loves their job? Of course not. But without them, factories would cease to exist. As would many of the things you take for granted every day: your car, your laptop, the sofa you're sitting on.

I say again: you don't have to love what you do for a living. *You just have to love your life.*

Maybe the assembly worker who fitted the door to your fridge loves being able to clock off at the same time every day and go home to his kids while it's still light outside. Maybe he loves the people he works with or the guaranteed overtime pay. He might not have grown up dreaming about staring at fridge doors all day, but it doesn't mean his life is any less fulfilling than yours.

This is another of those things I only really figured out when I thought I was going to the big boardroom in the sky. I, like a lot of people when they're diagnosed with cancer, had one of those terribly clichéd life-flashes-before-your-eyes moments. Only it doesn't flash exactly, like the film montages would have you believe. It just sort of ekes out slowly, like sap coming out of a tree, all viscous and surrounded by scar tissue. And I didn't find myself agonising over the things I thought I would. Not once did I think, 'How will I write that screenplay now?' Or, 'I never got to start my own homewares line.' In fact, work – real or imagined – didn't really factor into it at all. Other than the small fraction of time I lamented all those hours I'd spent worrying about invoices getting paid, but that was as deep as that well went.

Ask anyone who's dying and I dare say they'll have had the same insight. Work doesn't matter as much as we think it does when we're in the thick of it.

In terms of identity, you're no more your job than you are your hair colour. There are plenty of people out there who will judge you on both of these things, but a job title is no more a passport to happiness than dying your hair blonde. We can't all be TV presenters; we're not all going to be paid Instagram influencers – in fact, we can't even all afford to have a side hustle. But once more for the cheap seats: you don't have to have a hard-on for your work, you just have to be gratified with the life it affords you.

My dad was a great example. He worked for almost thirty years in a – I'm pretty sure he'd be okay with me saying this – reasonably mundane job. Monotonous, even. For decades he did the same thing, working mostly graveyard shifts and sleeping his days away. Then he retired – dreams of buying a beach house and watching his grandkids grow up quashed a year later when he was diagnosed with terminal lung cancer.

It sounds a bit morose, doesn't it? But while he probably didn't consider his humdrum government job was 'living his best life', I also don't think he'd go back and change it if given the chance. Because he worked that job, year in and year out, for us – his children. Working nights in a steady job meant our mother could work days, so someone was home for us twenty-four hours a day. We never wanted for anything, we were able to afford two family holidays a year and we don't have to look back on years spent in boarding school, with babysitters or at day care. We had parents who were always there for us. So while I'm quite sure my dad would have been more occupationally fulfilled writing science-fiction novels, I know he loved his life.

If you do happen to adore your job, then any itch you have to do more is probably just social media–induced anxiety getting the better of you. Go back to baking cakes/putting away bad guys/ training overweight bankers and take a moment to realise how lucky you are to be doing something you really, truly get a kick out of.

If you don't get much satisfaction out of your work, that's okay too. While you're thinking about what job you do want, just focus on the things you adore about your life. It's that simple.

That's what I did. Not because I don't love what I do, but because it mattered so little when I thought I was going to die. What mattered to me, what made my cup runneth over, was people. The people I cared about, the people who were looking after me, even people I hadn't met yet. That's what I yearned for more than anything – those relationships I now might never get to have. Because the mark you leave in this world isn't on a Wikipedia page, it's an ink stain on the hearts and minds of the people you have loved along the way. I realised work was really just a thing that afforded me the time and space to spend time with those people. All I really wanted to focus on going forward was *more people.*

Does it really take having your life threatened to come to this revelation? It did for me, but maybe it doesn't have to for you. Maybe you can be more like Dorothy and find your way back to Kansas without losing any of yourself in the process.

Paul White is a guy who found his way back to Kansas. Mostly because he lives there. He's a doctor, psychologist, speaker, author and general expert on workplace relations. He co-authored *The 5 Languages of Appreciation in the Workplace* with Dr Gary Chapman, of *New York Times*–bestseller fame *The 5 Love Languages.* Want to talk about toxic work culture? Paul's your guy. Want to talk about tornados with someone who has a lilting Midwestern accent? Paul's your guy. But we're really more interested in the first one because wanting to leave your job and needing to leave your job are worlds apart. Let's start by first figuring out which camp you're in.

'The core time to quit your job is when it's damaging your health – whether that's physical health, emotional health, relational health, spiritual health – when it's affecting you negatively, big time,' says Paul.

And the most telling warning sign?

'Commonly you're losing sleep,' says Paul. 'Which then sets up a whole chain of events that doesn't sit well. You're not exercising, you're gaining weight, you're drinking too much, you come home and just watch TV for hours or people tell you you're irritable all the time. When it starts to affect you to the point other people are noticing it, you better take a closer look. When something affects our wellbeing that significantly – to the point we're declining in health and even going towards illness – that's toxic. All these micro events of trauma add up to a toxic environment. I also know when

I say "toxic environment", a lot of people will picture this worker in a hazmat suit surrounded by chemicals, but it's any place you're being damaged or at risk of being damaged. If you continue on in that place, you'll suffer.'

And how do you know you're in one of these damaging cocoons exactly?

'There are really three key pointers to a toxic workplace,' says Paul. 'One is sick systems – in the sense the workplace isn't set up well as far as communication, decision-making, management and accountability. The five top toxic systems I found are hospitals, public schools, government social agencies, universities and colleges, and long-term care facilities. They're all serving multiple clients including families and insurance companies, and all have multiple reporting relationships. That creates confusion for everyone.

'Secondly, toxic leaders. A toxic leader is different than an incompetent one – at their core, a toxic leader is narcissistic. They'll take credit for other people's work, they'll shift blame – their decisions are always about what will make them look good and succeed, not what will make other people or the organisation succeed. They'll see people as just a resource to be used, like paper and staplers. One of the challenges of toxic leaders is that they often look good on paper at the beginning, otherwise they wouldn't have gotten the position. They can be very verbal, social and charismatic even. Rules don't apply to them, which makes them condescending.

'Then the third characteristic of a toxic workplace is dysfunctional colleagues. We're all dysfunctional to some degree, but these people often have dysfunctional health problems despite functioning in real life. Whether they can't maintain long-term relationships, they have financial problems, drug and alcohol abuse, anger issues, whatever it may be. What that looks like in the workplace is someone who doesn't take responsibility for their own actions; they're experts at blaming and making excuses. They're also big on indirect communication. They go around people, they send messages through people, they gossip, that kind of stuff.'

If you're nodding your head along to all of this like you're in a mosh pit circa 1996, then you may not just be in a job you don't like, you might be in one that's shortening your life. There's a pretty big chasm between not loving your job and working in a harmful job – so certainly mind the gap before you endure something that could actually be killing you. Wanting to leave a role because you don't like the amount of admin you have to do and being stressed to the point of developing anxiety are two very different things. If you're in the latter category you're not loving your job *or* your life, so it's time to jump ship. Don't even wait for the rescue boat – just hurl yourself in the calming waters of not-being-in-that-environment-any-more.

'The first step is taking care of yourself, because, if you don't, nobody will. You've got to set some boundaries. You've got to get some healthy habits into your life. Secondly, you also need to get some support. Toxic leaders control and manipulate and distort information, as do dysfunctional colleagues. When you're in a place like that, you're not even sure if you're thinking right or not. You need external support and counsel. It doesn't have to be professional, but I mean somebody who thinks straight, a sounding board. Someone you can bounce thoughts off. You need that support. It could be somebody within the system or it might just be a friend.'

One thing we have yet to really touch on is workplace trauma – because your great trauma may well be a professional one. And guess what – experts say you can get PTSD from work too.

'Trauma and PTSD tend to have a very intense connotation, but it can certainly exist in day-to-day life,' says Paul. 'Unpredictability is a big part of trauma. Think about a physically abusive father –

you never know if he's going to come home angry or not. It's unpredictable and that's traumatic in itself. Or in a war zone, you never know when a bomb's going to come raining down. One of the key things about mental health and dealing with it is predictability. And toxic leaders are unpredictable – one day you walk in and they're cheerful and warm, then maybe later that day they just tune you out like nobody's business. Unpredictability will put you on edge all the time. What even happens to some people is over a long period of time something becomes intense enough to be considered a disorder. When you call something a disorder, it means it's really negatively impacting your life in a significant way, different than a challenge or a problem. If you have a situation that's really intense, it's happening all the time, and then you add unpredictability in there as well – its effects will be felt in all areas of your life.'

So you know what – as much as you might loathe them – if you're in a toxic workplace, go ahead and stick up as many motivational quotes as you can find if that's going to help you extract yourself from a place more noxious than a sulphur mine in high summer. If this is akin to your situation, you probably *do* need to make your passion your profession – assuming you have a passion for not being treated like a bug on the windshield of life.

Everyone else: you're still not going to be discovered by a Hollywood talent agent while buying milk. Move on.

What each and every one of us needs, though, is good professional relationships. Because just like everywhere else in life, people matter. And Paul, of course, can tell you exactly what that looks like.

'There's been a shift recently around workplace culture in terms of relationships being important. The nature of work has changed so much – we're processing so much data and information, and for a while we forgot to make room for relationships. You had Uber falling apart because they were only focused on profit, then

Google had the issue with the guy who wrote that memo about sexism and stereotyping – so in Silicon Valley right now there's a really big emphasis on workplace culture. The understanding is it's not only about productivity. And the flipside is it's not just about relationships, either – we're not just going to work to have a good time. But we're finally getting to an understanding that you need a healthy relational workplace for good work to get done.'

When I first got sick, I avoided telling my publishers and editors. Basically: I didn't want to rock the relationship. I didn't want them to think I wouldn't be up to the job or, worse still, to just replace me with someone else. But once that was no longer viable, I had to act pretty quickly lest they found out from someone else. So I wrote them a long email detailing my sticky position and proactively thanking them for being so great and understanding and providing such amazing publications for me to work on. I went all in. And all that anxiety about being ousted just fizzled out. Because I was leaning on the relationships we had forged over several years to make the whole situation as nontoxic as possible. And those editors were largely pretty great about it. Okay, there was that one who basically never spoke to me again, but a pox on her house. That's just life. Everyone else rolled with it like a boss. Which is fitting, since that's what they were.

Now try this: write your work wife a thank-you note

If you don't have a work wife, then pen a memo to your boss, client, employee or partner. It doesn't have to be about anything grand or dramatic, just a written appreciation of their role in your everyday. Whether you're in this job for a good time, a long time or just until you find out you're the Crown Princess of Genovia, it's about trust.

'Trust is the foundation of all relationships,' says Paul. 'It's one of the key lessons a baby has to learn, in fact. If when they cry they don't know if anybody's going to respond, some babies actually just learn to give up. Because trust has to do with predictability and security. It's why economies like that of Russia in the '90s was so screwed up – because nobody followed through with commitments. People overseas would make orders, let's say, for steel or parts and then it wouldn't arrive in the agreed-upon quality. In any work relationship, if they don't follow through on what they say, you can't do business with them.

'One model I like to give people is built on that of the three Cs. Competence: can you do the job or task you're assigned. Consistency: do you show up, do you do it regularly, do you follow through and so forth. And character: do you take into account others' needs as well as your own. If you're missing any one of those, you're going to be a difficult person to trust.'

So be present, be involved – you don't have to heart your job, but you do have to do it to the best of your abilities. Being good at your job is also a pretty good indicator that you'll be more fulfilled in other areas of your life too. Work is not in a separate box that you close the lid on when you go home. All the areas of your life are moving parts of the same machine, a bicycle shaped uniquely like you. Put too much emphasis on one part and it will be to the disservice of the others.

Amazon CEO Jeff Bezos once described the relationship between his work life and personal life as being reciprocal. 'It's actually a circle. It's not a balance,' he said. In other words, it's not about trading off one thing for another; rather, it's about each thing being integrated and feeding into each other in a big rainbow-coloured loop.

Paul agrees with this sentiment. 'It's not all cut-and-dried compartmentalisation. And life seem to work best when there's some overlay – as that pertains to work, it means you may have some relationships you enjoy at work or you socialise with your colleagues,' he says.

What you do have to be careful about is neglecting your personal life in favour of your job. Checking work emails at your daughter's birthday party probably isn't going to make you a better parent, or even employee. But recognising that the lines are blurred and making that work to your advantage, by creating a work environment that benefits your health, will. The amount of emotional energy we spend on work is perhaps a little out of proportion in this day and age, with side hustles and crowdfunding and personal brands – it's a lot to take on for anyone. So again I say, make sure that effort is spread out over your life and don't put too much pressure on yourself to 'succeed'. Because when you get to your deathbed, you won't measure that success in award statues and degrees; *you'll measure it in relationships*. I can all but promise you that.

Idolising the work that other people are doing – or that you think they're doing – is never going to lead to a good place. Stop slavishly slobbering on motivational memes and get on with the business of just spending your time well out here in the real world. Even the guy whose work is based on other people's work agrees with me. And he's working on work to the power of two.

'I call it the California approach to career direction: that idea of finding what you love and going for it,' says Paul. 'But you know what – that's not the way the world works. You can't just be anything you want – there are limitations. Life limitations, personal limitations. A career is a pathway; you're walking a path and you make decisions along the way. You learn what you're good at and you follow that fork in the road. Almost every entry-level job sucks in some way. It's either low pay, bad hours, boring, dangerous, in a bad part of town, with bad customers, something's not great. But we all have to start there. That's partly why we have such a high dissatisfaction rate, because we've created such unrealistic expectations about work.'

Don't stay in a poisonous job, but don't feel bad about not having a business idea to submit to *Shark Tank* either. When someone asks you what you want to achieve in life, your answer should be something like: 'To have great relationships. To inspire people. To be inspired. To be happy and live long enough to see at least seven or eight decades around the sun.'

When you're spending a third of that time at work, you certainly want it to be a good third. Just don't let the other two thirds languish like fish on a pier.

The trick to all of this, of course, is having the confidence to know what you want most in life. Which means not only knowing your strengths but also acknowledging your weaknesses. Something we can work out over pizza, if you're keen?[1]

---

1   The next chapter involves pizza. Lots of pizza.

CHAPTER SEVENTEEN

Ty and Jay

(Or: How to cultivate confidence)

There is ample evidence that a lifestyle based on healthy eating and a little exercise is basically the $40 million Powerball of life. You'll sleep better, stave off umpteen diseases, find yourself less depressed and even live longer. The one unfortunate side effect, as far as I can tell, is that it makes us feel really bad about eating pizza, and for the longest time I found indulging in a pepperoni special to be a terrible, guilt-inducing act. It was almost as if by ordering a pizza on a Friday night, I was somehow disappointing both past Emma and future Emma simultaneously. That I was both ruining work that had already been done and hampering forthcoming efforts all at the same time. Reaching for that third slice felt like punching myself in the face for all the good it would do to my appearance and mood and demeanour, was my general analysis. I'd chastise myself for being weak and make a promise I'd never order takeaway again, knowing full well I didn't mean it even while wiping the grease from my fingers.

But those days are over – which is not to say I eat any more or less pizza than I did before; I've just learned not to make myself feel like an awful person for craving stuffed crust. This is no mean feat given the standards we hold ourselves up to in this life – the expected specs of beauty and success that are tenderised into tiny pieces and imbedded in our psyche early in life. Not to say anything about willpower, that oft celebrated but essentially non-existent trait we seem to hold so dear. Well, screw that. Life really is too fleeting to not appreciate the majesty of a short-order cook.

As I see it, this is essentially a spin-off of confidence. And I don't mean the 'forget the number on the tag, I'm wearing this bikini anyway' kind of confidence. I mean the 'if it all ended today, I wouldn't have any regrets' confidence. The variety you only get from well and truly being at peace with your place in the world.

Think about the most admirably confident person you know. The one with so much self-love, it oozes out of their pores. The one who laughs so hard, the people at the next table turn and stare, or who pulls off hats that would make most people more self-conscious than a Catholic priest at a gay pride parade. I guarantee you right now that person doesn't expend any energy feeling guilty about eating pizza. These people are well aware of their weaknesses, pizza cravings included; they just choose to work on their self-esteem instead of their self-doubt.

Allow me this opportunity to tell you a little bedtime story ...

There once was a boy named Ty (that's not his real name, but how baller are two-letter names?). Anyway, it's fair to say Ty didn't have a great time at school. He developed a stutter, got bullied and found himself drowning socially and academically. He learned very quickly just how mean kids could be. He felt like an outcast. He was depressed. He fell deeper and deeper into that well, to the point that he felt he was just flailing wildly without anywhere to turn.

Meanwhile, across country, there was another boy. This one was named Jay (also not his real name, but that three-letter blandness really drives my point home). Jay was a little older than Ty, but found himself similarly afflicted. He also raged against a speech impediment, well into adulthood in fact. An experience he describes as both desperate and embarrassing. Jay, just like Ty, was teased mercilessly for his stutter.

Ty and Jay would eventually meet, but that wouldn't happen for a while.

Still, their stories seemed to follow a similar trajectory. Neither ever had any professional help for their perceived weaknesses; instead, they just took it upon themselves to work on their confidence. Ty took some acting classes and Jay learned to recite poetry. Both were simply attempting some form of self-improvement; just trying to lift themselves out of the societal rut in which they found themselves in any way they could. Both, very gradually, learned that if you try hard enough, you can use your weakness to your advantage.

Ty and Jay eventually grew into adults with careers and families. Both were considered successful – role models even. But neither forgot about what it was like to have their weaknesses used against them.

It wasn't until almost four decades later that the pair finally met. On stage, as it happens, at the American Institute for Stuttering's annual gala. Both Ty and Jay spoke about how using acting and poetry to control their stutter led them to be the men they are today, to the careers they now enjoy, to the life they now love. How overcoming their stutter taught them to be the best public speakers they could be. How they fostered their self-confidence until their strength shouted louder than their fragility.

These are men who didn't just turn their weaknesses into an advantage, they beat them into submission and fed on the remains.

Ty and Jay are far better known as action hero Bruce Willis and former Vice President of the United States Joe Biden, respectively. And they're examples shinier than a couple of brand new Teslas. Men so confident it not only oozes out of their pores, but all over the headlines. What's worth noting is that they didn't set out to work on their weaknesses, specifically. Acting and poetry recital were obviously helpful for the stuttering, but it was their self-confidence they were trying to cultivate. And because they spent time polishing it so explicitly, it paid dividends.

This is something a lot of people simply don't do. If you want biceps that would put Aquaman to shame, you work on them daily – maybe every second day if you're going for more of a Ryan Gosling look. But you know full well it's going to need regular dedication. Self-confidence is much the same – it grows with attentiveness, but atrophies with neglect. So here's how you practise self-confidence.

Now try this: order a pizza

1) I told you pizza was coming! So buy yourself your favourite circle-based treat and, while you tuck into your first slice sans guilt, literally make a list of your weaknesses.

For example, my weaknesses include, but are not limited to:

- Terrible with money.
- Not great at saying no.
- Eats all the cheese in the fridge when left home alone.
- Lies about exercising when people ask.
- Gets jealous when my friends make new friends.
- Absolutely useless at asking for help.
- Once stole money from my mum's purse.
- Also from my dad's wallet. (Yes, I know. See item one.)

Seeing your many weaknesses all laid out in black and white like that might seem like a confronting exercise. But knowing what they are makes you far less flawed, ironically. Because everyone has them. Superman has kryptonite, Dracula has sunshine, Leonardo DiCaprio has women and you've got yours. Knowing them hopefully means you won't let them get out of hand.

As you look at them, you might also notice how subjective they are. Are you *actually* terrible at maths, or did you just decide that when you failed that one maths test when you were fifteen and you've been going with it ever since? You run this life – don't ever take gospel from your teenage self. Fifteen-year-old you also probably thought smoking was cool and 'groupie' was a valid occupation. They're really not much of an authority here. Facing your weaknesses is the first – and possibly most important – step to hyper confidence.

2) Pick up a second slice and decide if you're lucky.

Because you may or may not be.

Of course, there's a catch – because while luck exists, we make our own. Yes, that's a real thing. Don't worry – once again I have science on my side to prove it.

A psychologist named Richard Wiseman (if his nickname isn't Clever Dick, it really should be) did a ten-year study on luck and discovered 'lucky' people smile twice as often as 'unlucky' people. They also make more eye contact and are more extroverted. Unlucky people, poor sods, conversely scored far higher on neuroticism in the same study. What was Clever Dick's conclusion? That people who self-labelled themselves as lucky increased their opportunities because they were more observant, met more people and maintained better relationships. On the flipside, he found anxiety tends to blind us to opportunities – as such, self-professed unlucky people missed out on things because they were too busy worrying about ... well, other things.

Luck, therefore, is largely something you fertilise. And lucky people will always be self-confident people. So open your eyes – luck no more eludes you than the spare sunglasses that are in your glove compartment. You're here and that already makes you luckier than the other 99 million-odd sperm that didn't make it. Double chin up, people.

3) Reach for a third and call a friend.

This one is so key to self-confidence, it's practically hanging on a chain from your ignition. Your friendships are the absolute best mental buffer you have. Cherish them, coddle them, do not take them for granted.

I don't care if you only have one solitary pal – call them and tell me you don't feel better for it. Quality over quantity on this front. We're talking the type of people who will hold your hair back when you're throwing up after your fourteenth round of chemo. How many people would you trust to do that? If you can count five, you're already living your best life. It mightn't seem it, especially considering you're now hypothetically vomiting up toxic substances, but you really are. The reason I think this is twofold.

First fold: Almost every single time someone pontificates about self-confidence, it's as an introspective exercise. Visualise a more confident you, do daily affirmations, identify your talents. So few top-line suggestions have anything to do with other people. But if you don't have friends wiping away your tears and cheering your successes, any gains will feel pretty hollow. A good friend will always be able to pump you up when you accidentally leave your optimism on the top of the car and it flies off like an errant cappuccino. Nothing is better for your self-confidence than that.

Second fold: Friends are so important to your self-worth, a recent study showed eating meals alone to be the biggest single factor dictating unhappiness behind an existing mental illness. People who spend time sharing meals with friends are simply happier people. We have no idea why. We just know the social act itself releases endorphins, which are chemically similar to opioids. So sharing a feed with a pal will literally give you a high. We're biologically engineered to feed off each other's very presence, so if you need to work on your self-confidence, stop trying to do it alone. Studies show a minimum of three face-to-face social interactions a week will help give you that buzz.

4) Eat the rest of your pizza, recycle the box and scare the living bejesus out of yourself.

Being confident has nothing to do with not being scared; they're not mutually exclusive in any way. Fear is actually an incredibly important tool for getting you to where you need to go, both physically and metaphorically. Were Bruce and Joe pooping their bloomers the first time they tried reciting something on stage? You bet. But they practised it over and over until they could do it with the whole world watching.

Pushing through fear is flipping terrifying – not least of which because our bodies are hardwired to think we're going to die if we don't succeed. That the lion will eat us or the rock avalanche will crush us. In the twenty-first century, however, the worst that will happen is we might have to take a job as a waiter. Probably worth the punt.

I punched through the fourth wall of my confidence just as I finished treatment. A mentor of mine decided it was time for me to be back up on stage. But even having been a comedian for almost a decade, I found the idea of doing stand-up post-chemo quite terrifying. I had always joked about dating and drama; now I was suddenly supposed to switch to needles and nurses. Not to mention I'd be doing it bald and in a mastectomy bra, without even a single eyelash to combat the bright lights and expectant faces. I had no idea how the audience would cope.

It took a lot of convincing, but I did it. Some people squirmed, others laughed, some even thanked me afterwards. I had been so petrified of freaking other people out, I couldn't see past my own ego. It had nothing to do with being bald and everything to do with being afraid. But it turns out I could be humorous and tumorous at the same time, and to great effect. And to think ... I was once afraid of a pizza.

Confidence is doing things for *you*, not for some imaginary audience you've allowed to mill around in your frontal lobe. It's not, 'Everyone will like me when I'm charismatic and charming.' It's simply, 'I've got this whether they like me or not.' And it's worth the pursuit. Confidence is more satisfying than knowing you're going to finish the shampoo and the conditioner at the same time, every time. It will see you through trauma with grace, style and one hell of an attitude. So, go – do something that scares you. Try rock climbing, call that friend you haven't spoken to in a year, wear pink.

I honestly try to do something that scares me every day. Some days it's as simple as sending an email or squashing a spider (sorry ... animals were definitely harmed in the making of this book) – other times it's more gargantuan, like moving countries or letting my sister do my eye makeup. What scares you will be a whole different bowl of nuts, but avoiding those things is like living your whole life inside a freezer. There's the quiet life and there's an indistinguishable life. You do not want the latter. But build your confidence enough and trauma won't be able to touch the sides.

What will touch you, however, is what I have for you in the next chapter. It will quite literally touch you in places you didn't even know you could be touched. Intriguing? Absolutely.

CHAPTER EIGHTEEN

Netflix & Pills
(Or: The weird world of
sensory stimulation)

Humans have a pretty remarkable ability to adapt to things. Not hawkfish-level remarkable, mind you – those things can change sex and back again whenever it suits them. We're dullards compared to that. But we adapt to things more readily than most of us probably imagine.

The most compelling part is that this malleability works both ways. We can adapt frighteningly quickly to pleasant things – like that car we saved up for or that job we really wanted. They're fun at first, but the joy fades fast and then it's on to the next thing. But we can get acclimatised to unpleasantries with breathtaking momentum as well.

If you've ever found yourself in a situation where people say the phrase 'I can't even imagine what you're going through' around you, then you probably already know this. Whether that position was finding yourself presented with an awful prognosis, having someone you love involved in an accident or being a party to a divorce you didn't see coming. At first, it's like a pipe bomb has gone off in your life – shrapnel pierces you from all directions and you cry out for help that might never come. After a while, though, it becomes part of you. Whether you like it or not. It goes from being an imaginable horror to something you have to integrate into your everyday life.

This transition is more difficult for some people than it is for others. There are some that get stuck in a feedback loop they can't get out of; the pain is just as raw months later as it was when it first happened. For these people, nothing anyone says or does makes much difference. There is no external stimulus louder than the internal monsoon.

If that sounds like you, here are three phrases I'd like you to completely ignore from now on. Don't heed them, don't believe them and definitely don't say them to anyone else. Let me break down why these are the most obnoxious idioms to give someone who's struggling.

a) Everything happens for a reason
The implication that someone's heinous misfortune is for a greater good is actually quite outrageous. The world is chaos and that's okay. It doesn't mean there's a master plan for your torment.

b) I guess it wasn't meant to be
You're essentially saying to someone they weren't destined to have a good life. So that's pretty offensive, isn't it?

c) God only gives you what you can handle
To start with, not everyone believes there is a God. So you could possibly correct this to: 'Humans have an amazing ability to deal with what life throws at them.' That doesn't make it any easier to handle at the time, though.

I would like to call bullshit on these and every other ridiculously unhelpful saying people fling at you when shit goes down. But more to the point, if you are still struggling months after a crisis, please get some counselling. There is absolutely nothing on this planet that anyone should have to go through alone and certainly not for any significant length of time. There are some things a flimsy book just won't touch. If you're not quite ready to seek out a professional just yet, allow me to suggest the most glorious and slavish action of the modern age ... sending an email. Pick anyone you like: your brother, a friend, someone you haven't seen since high school – just reach out, see how they are and tell them what you've got going on. Even that level of human contact will be useful for your beaten spirit. Souls are a lot like peaches – easily bruised but covetable nonetheless. Don't let yours wither more than it has to.

Those cases aside, most of us will be adapters, for better or worse. And there are several ways in which this adaptation can be exploited as a strength. Take jet lag, for example – our body's way of adjusting to the fact there's a new time sheriff in town. While we tend to feel this disturbance to our natural rhythms keenly at first, our bodies will eventually acclimate. Coffee, sunlight, melatonin – whatever helps you bridge that gap, you use it. But in the end your body finds its way.

Dealing with trauma is not unlike forcing your body into a new time zone. When we struggle with a trauma, we're learning to adapt to something on a higher emotional level. It takes longer and it's far more complicated – but it's a similar process. And whatever you need to get you through, that's what you do.

For instance, my body really struggled to adapt to sleep post mastectomy. I was always a stomach sleeper, you see. Mad for it. I've just always found it more comforting to have my face, chest, genitals and other important parts of me squished into the mattress where they couldn't come to any harm overnight. But there's nothing like open-chest surgery to really put a crimp in that sort of style.

For months I had to sleep like I was perpetually flying in economy. Not quite flat, not quite upright, always facing forward and about as frustrated as a fly in a jar. As my wounds started to heal, I attempted to graduate into a side sleeper, but that was no less painful than sticking rusty nails up my nostrils.

We need sleep like we need oxygen – yet while we wouldn't willingly deprive ourselves of oxygen for hours at a time, many of us do this with sleep day after day. Especially when we're going through trauma. But if our most base needs aren't being met, it's very hard to work on anything more intellectual. Our adaptation gets halted at the most basic level.

Several months of Netflix and pain pills later, and I was back in hospital, complaining to a particularly conscientious nurse about the fact I couldn't sleep, yet again. I was living in the moderate hope that he'd give me a little somethin'-somethin' to take the edge off. A tiny tablet or two that would gently push me over the cliff of consciousness. But having recently bonded over a shared love of *Star Trek* and mint-flavoured chocolate, it seemed he felt our bond had matured to the point of personal – because he paused slightly before letting me in on a little secret. Something for which I will always be grateful. Not as grateful as I am for the several times he had to lift me onto a bedpan so I could relieve myself, but it's up there.

'You want to try something a little crazy?' he said.

'Yeah, whaddya got?' I said, thinking I might get the *really* good stuff if I played it cool.

'It's a blanket ...' he said, teasingly.

Really? A blanket? I was exhausted to the point of hallucinating, and he was suggesting a blanket. I could have kneecapped him.

'Yeah, I use it all the time,' he went on. 'I have mine in my car downstairs actually. It's heavy – like, really heavy. Do you want to try it?'

'Sure,' I said, finally understanding. It was *heavy*, man. The blanket was a ruse after all. A way for him to surreptitiously slip me some mind-bending pills under the covers without the hospital cameras catching on. I was totally picking up what he was putting down.

Turns out it really was just a blanket. I was more deflated than my own left breast.

He placed it on top of me gingerly but adeptly, like a pastry chef throwing a layer of fondant over a wedding cake.

'What do you think?' he asked.

Wow, did I feel like a jerk. Not only did my nurse have exquisite taste in science fiction, he was sharing his own personal comforter with me. And it was just that – an object more comforting than drowning in a litter of chinchillas. It wasn't disconcerting, it wasn't something I had to get used to – it was instantly consoling. And he was right – it was *heavy*. I could finally sleep on my back and still feel like all my squishy pink bits were safe from bumps in the night.

My night nurse had introduced me to the weird world of weighted blankets.

What is a weighted blanket, exactly? It's what it says on the tin, to be honest – it's a heavy blanket. But not like 1200-thread-count heavy, like *medicinally* heavy. Up to ten kilos or more.

It's not a new idea by any means – over the years, weighted blankets have been used to treat patients ranging from anxious puppies to children living with autism. But they've enjoyed a pop-culture surge recently thanks in part to their use as an under-the-counter treatment regime for soldiers returning home with PTSD from our current slew of incursions. The research on this is still in its infancy at best – but anecdotally, it works wonders for a lot of people. Not everyone, but a lot.

And the best part about a blanket as opposed to say, an opioid, is that if it doesn't float your particular yacht, there are almost zero side effects. In a world where pharmaceutical addiction is a very real problem, I wanted to know more about this mysterious shroud. Turns out cavewomen and rats are our teachers on this one.

Well, cavewomen, rats and deep pressure stimulation.

'Deep pressure stimulation is really any type of tactile input that's designed to be deep as opposed to superficial. So if you can imagine someone running a feather along your arm, or lightly tickling you – that's superficial touch. Deep touch would be somebody coming along and putting their hands on your shoulders and pushing down, or giving you a massage even. Things that are stimulating those deep tactile receptors.'

That's the erudite utterance of one Stacey Reynolds. Stacey is a PhD-toting associate professor and occupational therapist with Virginia Commonwealth University. She knows a *lot* about neuroscience and sensory processing. But let's get to the cavewomen and the rats.

'We know that light touch is alerting to the sympathetic nervous system, to our fight-or-flight mechanisms – so our body is sent into high arousal, physiologically, by light-touch stimulation,' she says. 'And we think that's probably evolutionary – if you were a cavewoman asleep and something brushed by you, you're going to need to be alerted immediately. Whereas if you were in that same situation but you had a crying baby, you'd need to calm that baby down, otherwise the tiger that brushed by you before is going to find you and eat you. And so mothers hold their babies to comfort them; they use swaddles and the like to stop the crying, to protect the family. This is all conjecture, but it explains how light touch might increase arousal while deep touch reduces arousal.'

And the rats?

'Well, there's this guy named Michael Meaney; he did a lot of rat research. The punchline of what he found was that the more touch the rat pups received – particularly mothers licking and grooming their pups – the better the pups dealt with stress their entire lives. So that early licking and grooming behaviour set those pups up to deal with stressors their entire life. And they were able to trace that back to brain receptors – their brains had more receptors for a chemical called cortisol, a stress hormone. In those rats, the cortisol would bind to the stress receptors and shut that stress response off faster, because they had that early stimulation.'

So deep pressure touch = feeling safe. Whether it's because our cavewoman ancestors held us to their bosom or not, we don't know. We just know it works. Something I can attest to from that super snug feeling I got in the hospital. Not something one usually associates with beds in wards.

But it's not just blankets that have this effect. Stacey did an entire study just on vests.

'It was a deep pressure vest that used a balloon-type material, as opposed to just heavy weights,' she says. 'Some trends we found from the research were that people would opt to wear it before they went to a social event they might normally find anxiety inducing, as a preparatory activity. Some also said it would be helpful before a job interview. So those were the kind of situations we thought would be useful in adults.

'With children – especially autistic children – parents are really looking for things that will help them at school. We envisioned that kids may be able to wear the vest during test-taking, or again as a preparatory thing. Even that kids could have objects like these in an area in the classroom they could go to when they were stressed – they might have the option to use a vest, or a blanket, or they could get under a heavy pillow or mattress.

'Then of course there's a lot of research that's been done into things like massage as an intervention, or hold positions that a mother might use in the NICU with a small baby to instigate a calming effect. Other objects that have been used therapeutically are things like weighted lap blankets.'

So it's a whole academic thing, this whole pin-yourself-under-overweight-objects malarkey.

It's not just any old heavy object, though. A weighted blanket, for example, should sit at around ten per cent of your body weight. You may perhaps expect you'd find that claustrophobic, but it's really just shades of being tucked in as a child or having someone you love fall asleep on top of you. Someone who's actually incredibly light and you don't have to shove off after twenty minutes.

Studies have shown some people even fall asleep faster and sleep more deeply under a weighted blanket. And, as you can imagine, there's far less tossing and turning. The general rub is the body experiences an evenly distributed sensory pressure which may naturally decrease your heart rate and blood pressure. In that way, it promotes completely drug-free relaxation, ergo a sleep deeper than an Adele album. Some of Stacey's results even pointed towards the fact that deep pressure stimulation might help increase attention to a task.

'The results aren't totally clean, but children with ADHD were making fewer errors with the application of deep pressure. Our theory behind that is that if we can reduce their physiological arousal, they're going to be able to focus their attention, as opposed to being anxious and vigilant about everything,' says Stacey. 'But there are definitely links between arousal and anxiety levels because when you're in high arousal you're also increasing your vigilance – you're scanning your whole environment to look for threats. But when you're physiologically calm and focused, you're able to decide what you want to pay attention to – as opposed to feeling like you need to be on alert to everything that's going on.'

While the jury might still be out on weighted blankets, scientists can in fact measure this fierce arousal with a startling degree of accuracy. And if you just giggled at the phrase 'fierce arousal' then we can be friends.

'The three ways most people do this, including us, is to look at three different systems: the sympathetic and the parasympathetic system, which together are known as the autonomic nervous system; then the third is looking at neuro-endocrine activity.'

So let's just buy that idea a drink and get to know it a little better, shall we …

Basically the sympathetic system is our fight-or-flight response, the parasympathetic system is the complete opposite (also sometimes called our 'rest-and-digest response'), and neuro-endocrine activity is what the brain does with all the hormones flying around in there.

'So I mentioned cortisol earlier,' says Stacey. The rats, remember? 'That's the primary neuro-endocrine hormone that people look at to measure stress. So when something occurs, your body produces this stress hormone, which helps mobilise your body to deal with it. And then the cortisol goes back up to the brain and says, "Hey, this stress has been dealt with, shut-off time." So cortisol basically works on this feedback loop, and there are a lot of conditions where that loop gets broken – if you get too much cortisol in your system it will stop working. PTSD and depression are the two most famous conditions where this happens.'

It's like an iPhone that's been dropped down the stairs too many times – at some point the home button just stops working.

'We also look at galvanic skin response, which measures electrical conduction of the skin through sweat gland activity,' says Stacey. 'It's what lie detector tests use. The whole premise of those is if you're going to tell a lie, you're going to have a change in arousal before you do it, and we can pick this up by measuring the sweat gland activity on the palm of your hand. It's a similar thing here.'

So while there might not be enough evidence for your medical insurance to swing you a weighted blanket for what ails ya, the research in this field is pretty exciting.

Overall, what deep pressure stimulation seems most effective for is anxiety. It was only after my nurse turned me into a brick chicken I realised how anxious those post-surgical nights made me. The more I couldn't sleep, the more I'd be anxious about not sleeping. Talk about a feedback loop.

And anxiety is something we all have to some degree. Especially when we're stressed, whether that be physically or mentally.

War vets are a great example. A lot of veterans experience sleep disorders, including insomnia and night terrors, after they return from active duty, so weighted blankets were touted as an answer to a more restful night's sleep. The PTSD they experience is often a complex melange of the physical, mental and emotional, and, for some, this type of device may actually offer blanket relief. Pun admittedly intended. Anecdotal evidence suggests some veterans find them to be a literal life saver.

As Stacey warns, though, they're not just a magical coverall.

'It's potentially very exciting, but worth noting that for some people, wearing a deep pressure vest may actually bring the trauma to the surface. This is the danger in just picking something up off the shelf – you want to make sure it isn't bringing back any type of negative feelings. Think about a deep massage you might have had in the past – it was probably a great massage, but sometimes you walk away and feel your mood has changed. Sometimes even in a negative direction. Deep pressure touch is just so powerful. But we know tactile stimulation can change the brain so I think there are definitely possibilities for using something like this either on a daily basis or in response to an acute stressor.'

Now try this: change your heart rate

One of the biggest indicators of autonomic arousal – whether it's going up or down – is heart rate. Where something like a weighted blanket will generally bring your heart rate down, something like watching a horror movie might bring it way up. A daily dose of blankie was my jam, but because we're all as individual as our fingerprints suggest, you have to figure out what your weighted quilt is. Is it compression tights? Silk sheets? The thing which nudges your arousal buttons might not actually be an object at all.

'Putting a weighted blanket on your lap is actually a very passive thing to do,' says Stacey. 'And it's not right or wrong, but it's very passive. When I work with kids, I also like to explore active ways to modify their arousal. So engaging in some type of heavy work task, where they're lifting, or pushing, or pulling; they're exercising. Or it might be something where they're engaging with other people.

'In occupational therapy, we talk a lot about a sensory diet. We try to train people to think about what they need to do every day to manage their arousal levels, to manage their anxiety in non-pharmacological ways. And most of us already engage in some type of sensory diet – some people need to run first thing in the morning, some people need to go to a fitness class at the end of the day to burn off steam, they need to fidget in class, or they need to do yoga. We all have things we do to manage our arousal levels. So ideally most adults would be able to understand their own physiology – they'd be able to think what times of day are most challenging for me, what situations are the most difficult? And then, what strategies can I develop to prepare myself for those situations and use to decompress afterwards?'

A weighted blanket was my way of adapting to a strange, new world. It might be yours too. Or your acclimatisation might take the form of Pilates or a white noise machine. Whatever it is, it will be something you can work into your everyday.

'The brain needs to integrate sensory information in order to have optimal functioning. And there are several studies out there that show this. People who have had environmental deprivation – kids who've grown up in orphanages, for example – have a lot of sensory integration problems. Because you learn to integrate your senses through engagement and practice in your environment. Eye–hand coordination is the best example of that. You don't just know how to catch a ball, you practise that. You repeat something over and over and your brain begins to link what you're seeing with what you're feeling, with what you're hearing, all the way through.'

This is the kind of repetitive diet I can get behind. With yoga and vests in place of egg-white omelettes and kale smoothies. Just like with any diet, results aren't always going to be instantaneous, but practice makes passable human beings.

If whatever you're going through is making you overtired, anxious, stressed – if you have trouble falling asleep or you wake up feeling as though you were attacked by rest-hungry vampires in your dreams – then working on your sensory diet will do wonders too. If you can't figure it out on your own, an occupational therapist can help. Once you get to this point, though – the point where you're not jumping out of your skin – we can move on to those head termites called emotions. So strap on your weighted vest and let's get down to business.

CHAPTER NINETEEN

Tiny little asshole dictators

(Or: Learning to corral your emotions)

When I was going through treatment, there were certain people who were astonished by how happy I seemed about the whole thing. And in trying to figure out why I was able to hold it together where other people couldn't, I realised perhaps the difference was in how I treat my emotions. I tend to think of them as being a lot like toddlers – tiny little asshole dictators bent on destroying all that is peaceful in the world.

No, I jest! Mostly.

But take a minute to think about toddlers – they're emotional explosions personified. Human-shaped volcanos of passion. They can be literally quivering with elation one minute only to be sobbing with grief the next. They don't yet have the cognitive ability to distil their feelings and as a result they all come tumbling out in real time. Completely unpredictable, utterly unfiltered.

The first time I was privy to such a haemorrhage of hysteria, I was babysitting my twenty-month-old nephew, Harry. He'd always been a very pleasant baby; a real giggle monster whose favourite things in life were blueberries and the moon. Babysitting him usually involved reading *Hairy Maclary* nine times in a row and maybe watching an episode of *Peppa Pig*. It was a sweet gig.

This particular day – a warm summer's afternoon – we'd just come home from lunch. Harry's parents were at work and I'd offered to hang out with him for the day in an effort to punch in a few hours on the favourite-aunt clock. I unbundled him from the car and chased him about the front lawn for a while. One of his favourite games at the time was run-at-the-main-road-full-speed. The fact you'd have to drop anything you were carrying in from the car to scoop him up before he got run over by a passing motorist amused him greatly.

Eventually we made our way inside and I shut the door behind us. Which is when it happened … Like nothing I'd ever seen before, an absolute detonation of despair. As instantaneous and hard to avoid as a confetti cannon. The outpouring of agony he displayed at simply no longer being outside took me completely off guard.

I stared at him for a while in wonderment – you rarely see such a raw human reaction when you're not used to being around small people. It shocks you into the moment like little else can. Not in a pleasant way, I might add, but it's very effective nonetheless. Mindfulness brought on by meditating the insanity before you.

So what did I do? Well, as a non-parent … I just let him go outside again. It wasn't my job to enforce discipline or rules, I figured. As the cool aunt, he would get to go whatever he wanted on my watch.

Fifteen minutes later, I was once again done playing chicken and herded Harry back inside. Which is when it happened again. With possibly even more ferocity. Fascinating, I thought, that anyone can feel this intensely about something so seemingly benign. I stared at him as he flailed around at my feet. Tears were running down his face and his ears were turning red. He screamed in a way that made it sound like I was slapping his backside with a cheese grater. At one point, he even started hyperventilating, as if invisible hands were squeezing his tiny lungs from within.

As someone who's done some acting, I have to say it's a performance Benedict Cumberbatch would have trouble replicating. They should make auditions for all movies from now on simply attempting a toddler tantrum – you'd soon weed the blah from the Blanchetts.

To me, emotions are very similar. They beg for attention in the same way, are often illogical in the same way and are prone to monopolising your time in the same way. They are a 24-hour-a-day nuisance you love and loathe in equal measure.

And just like a toddler, you can't stop an emotion from erupting. Nor should you try. They're a big part of our survival mechanism. Trying to nullify an emotion is like trying not to have a digestive system. No amount of thinking-it-so will make it happen and you'd quite likely cease to exist without it.

So if you can't stop your emotions, surely the answer to not letting them dictate your mood is in how you react to them – in the same way that a carer's reaction to a toddler will likely direct their mood. So what's the best way to do that exactly?

We know a lot more about taming infants than we do about taming the brain, so perhaps a toddler whisperer will have some answers we can use. We already know that a lot of how we deal with trauma in later life is dictated by what happens to us when we're in early childhood, so how we deal with tantrums is likely a trauma goldmine in miniature.

Enter Tovah Klein, PhD, associate professor of psychology, director of the Barnard College Center for Toddler Development (which just so happens to be located on Broadway in New York City – an address I find very fitting for studying a bunch of tiny drama queens) and author of *How Toddlers Thrive*. She's also served as an adviser for *Sesame Street* and knows more about how to subdue toddler tantrums than just about anyone, anywhere. So I tell her my theory about emotions being akin to toddlers.

'Well ... at our worst self we are just sort of elevated young children,' she says.

I take that as her being sceptically on board with my hypothesis. But what I really want to glean from her is, how do we handle a frenzied toddler with feelings to burn?

'I often say to parents, the lighter you can keep this, and the more humour you can have, the better you'll get through it,' she says. 'And if you really want to build a confident child, you pick your battles carefully. Do you really care if they have to have the red cup? Maybe not. But you do care that they hold your hand crossing a street, right? So it's not a limitless free-for-all, but it really is a case of picking the appropriate battle – knowing where to put the limits in.

'And I'm always telling parents the way to really head it off is to say to them, "You're not going to like this," or "I've got bad news – one more time down the slide and then we gotta go home for dinner." That says to the child, "I understand the disappointment that's about to come." It's like if your friend calls and says, "I've got really bad news." You'll obviously counter with, "Oh no, what?" And she says, "I've got to cancel our dinner plans tomorrow." That warning helps soften the blow; lessens the impact.'

So: humour helps, pick your combats carefully, don't be afraid of setting them up for defeat. This pretty neatly encapsulates how I dealt with the uncomfortable period between cancer test and test result, when emotions were at an all-time high. I made boob jokes more often than Buzzfeed posts frivolous quizzes. I completely ignored the fact that months of treatment might mean I wouldn't be able to pay my rent and went shopping instead. I let myself prepare for the worst, putting all the flashing warning signs in place – *you could be dying, you know, get ready for them to blurt out you have six months to live.*

I treated my terror like a toddler in every way Tovah suggests. And it made the scariest week of my life far more bearable.

If you're going through a particularly bad divorce, you can see how all of these things would help immensely too. Picking your battles may mean recognising that you're sad enough to indulge in a pint of ice cream but not letting yourself be angry enough to key his car in the dead of night. Or perhaps not having ridiculous expectations is knowing you won't be over her in a week, a month or even a year. Be gentle with yourself and your emotions the way you would a toddler. Because you're just as fragile, truth be told.

Not all strong emotions come from something so dramatic, though. Sometimes they come from something as simple as being a little off kilter, a little out of sorts.

'There are some big triggers common to all toddlers – so a child who's hungry, a child who hasn't had enough sleep, a child who's been off schedule,' says Tovah. 'Young children like routine. Or just not being overwhelmed. Maybe it's a weekend where you went from a birthday party to a friend's house to the park – it's just too much. But then certain children have particular triggers as well. There's some children who don't do well in large settings with lots of people they don't know, for example.'

Sound like you after you had to go to three lots of Christmas drinks in one night? Or had to field why-aren't-you-married-yet interrogations from several aunts in a row? Sometimes your emotions are every bit as fragile as a rug rat. In predicting and quelling these eruptions, Tovah is well versed too.

'I would say two things are important. One is the before: the more routines people have at home, the easier life is. You're regulating them, helping them move from one thing to the next. Giving them a very simple explanation helps with that. You know, "We're going to get in the car and we're going to see grandma. Grandma is going to be home. Remember grandma has a dog?" Giving them some explanation is helpful. We also need to recognise that parent expectations are often way too high. Do I really want to go to that fancy restaurant for our family dinner when my child's been in a pretty grumpy phase recently? Can I really expect her to sit at that table? The other piece of this is understanding that tantrums are a normal part of development. So to know that anger is part of life, and helping children understand that they'll have feelings of happiness and sadness, and anger, and excitement, that all helps the child realise this is normal.'

So don't put yourself in a position where you know your emotions will go into overdrive (i.e. knowing your ex will be at that party), don't have ridiculous expectations (say, that he's going to clock you across the room and suddenly realise he's made a huge mistake) and above all know you're completely normal (yes, everyone's fantasised about the across-the-room thing at some point ... trust me).

For me, it was Harry's not-so-little display that rammed the point home. I realised adults can get just as irrationally angry that our toast fell on the floor or just as excited when someone we love gets home. Only we've self-installed something of a brain Brita filter. We are, for the most part, able to control how much of that emotion we share with the outside world. The emotion itself is still there, it's just muffled. So why the shield?

Again, our toddler whisperer has the goods.

'We live in a world where your life is on view. It's not just on view on the sidewalk that you're walking down, it's on view to the world. Somebody is always photographing it, putting it on social media. We live in a world of shame, so to speak, and as such tantrums are embarrassing. A tantrum is completely unsocialised. It's really the anger, I think, that scares people – it's intense and it's kind of primal, and at least in our culture and our society we're socialised to not have anger. Not just to not show it, but to not feel it. So here's a child in front of you expressing basically what we would like to express in return but can't. So that's very scary to adults. We're socialised to show certain emotions but not show others. We also have a lot of cognitive thinking abilities. We can think, "Okay, I'm getting upset, but I can't chew out the store clerk, so how am I going to handle this dispute?" Toddlers have none of that – zero.'

So along with the bigger and more capable brain we gain as we grow, which gives us other, more acceptable ways to deal with these things, we're shamed by society not to throw tantrums. Which, with the exception of certain celebrities and world leaders, is an expectation we largely adhere to. But underneath that, the emotions are still there, as raw as a fresh graze. The real issue toddlers have to deal with – something Tovah calls the 'hallmark of two-year-olds' – is the discovery of pride and shame.

'I always say shame is good,' she says. 'Shame keeps us human and keeps us connected. Why do you stop at a traffic light when there's no cars around? Why don't you shove the person in front of you? The shame of doing the wrong thing. Shame is what makes us be able to live among each other. So it's naturally a good thing, but to shame a child can be very harmful. It works against them learning autonomy and a sense of self. Shame is a very powerful emotional part of personal trauma. Shaming or scolding them tells them I can't count on this person.'

You can see how shaming your own emotions is going to work in a very similar way. They're every bit as primal and crude as a toddler. Feeling embarrassed about an emotional reaction is going to make you retreat back into yourself even further. You can't help feeling what you feel. Not ever. And there's no shame in that.

'Also, the less critical the parent is, the more the child is going to be open about revealing their worst side of self,' says Tovah. 'We all have a good side of self, that's very easy to share, and we all have a less desirable part of self that we tend to dislike or be ashamed of. If the child feels they can reveal both sides and knows they're going to be okay even in their worst moments, that they won't be rejected, the child learns to be reasonable over time.'

And here's a thing I think is particularly important – don't disregard them, ever. Not the toddlers and not your emotions.

'I think the main thing is that people not abandon the child. If a toddler is throwing a tantrum, you don't have to cajole them or try to make them happy – being present is enough. Where trust comes from is when a parent is accepting of the child after one of these kind of blow-ups – I call it the repair. So when a repair happens, a parent might say, "You were very upset and I know that," then give them a hug and continue with, "But I love you even when you're that upset." They come back together, they trust each other.'

Let's just play out that message – don't expect a two-year-old (or an emotion) to do anything other than what it knows how to do. It's pure feels. Your only recourse is to let the drama fade naturally. It's an entity dependent on you in almost every way, one that asks 'why' incessantly and never wants to go to sleep. But – most importantly – it's one that needs guidance and patience-threatening amounts of devotion. Because what it all boils down to – the crusty stuff left at the bottom of the pan when all the other stuff has evaporated – is fear.

'Fear is something that's inborn,' says Tovah. 'This is true even in children who have been raised in loving, accepting households, who have never experienced it. It's not as if they were abandoned and fear being abandoned again. It's just a very natural human tendency.'

It's that fear you've had your whole life, that's written into your DNA, that makes you afraid and nervous and anxious even when it makes no sense. It's that fear that stops you from doing most things. But if at first you don't succeed, try not to dwell on it for the rest of your life. Because at some point you will fail so spectacularly that you'll wonder if you can love/laugh/show your face in the office again. The trick is not getting stuck in the quagmire.

Now try this: watch an episode of *Toddlers & Tiaras*

If you haven't already, watch yourself an episode of *Toddlers & Tiaras* (a reality show which aired 2009 through 2016 but is a lesson for the ages). Heck, just watch three minutes. Everything I just said will make so much sense when you know what a proper Hollywood-emphasised toddler tantrum really, truly looks like at its most inflated.

Then imagine that going on in your head. Instead of crying and wailing and asking 'Why me?' next time a virulent emotion strikes, you'll be much more likely to just sit in the corner and read a magazine until the whole thing dies down. Metaphorically speaking. You're not going to be able to stop yourself from hearing the hysterics, but you should be able to stop yourself from getting completely lost in them. Because you can be both sad and optimistic at the same time if you think of them as individual things. Perhaps even as small children who can learn how to play nice if given enough direction.

It's also in this way that happiness becomes just another ingredient in the goulash. Not the goal, not the pot of gold at the end of a self-help rainbow, just another emotion that will pop in and out of your head when you least expect it, like a kid playing hide-and-seek. Know that and the search not only seems easier, but the finding of it almost becomes a natural side effect of being alive. Because you know it will show itself eventually. You learn to come to peace with the fact you'll be happy one minute, angry the next and melancholy the one after that. Like Tovah says, we're just big kids, elevated in inches and lessened in incense.

Happiness is and always will be the one emotion we want most of all, though; it's a truth as cosmically accepted as death, taxes and the deliciousness of melted cheese. Learn to do the above and you'll find happiness is almost the afterglow. The real manoeuvre is knowing the problem doesn't lie in the finding of your happiness at all.

What is it then?

Well, you'll need to buy my next book, *Playing Hide the Sausage with Happiness*, to find out. RRP$29.95 at all good bookstores and where thought-provoking reads are sold.

Jokes! You just have to turn to the next section. Because it's got the last ingredients you need for garnishing your wellbeing enchilada.

BUT FIRST! RED-HOT HUMANITY HACKS: WHAT HAVE WE LEARNED?

That there's a lot of joy to be had in nature and other people. That on occasion you're probably being a bit of an ass-monkey yourself. That you need time-outs and perspective and pizza. That both your body and brain will sometimes need a little help from their friends. That your life isn't always going to smell like fart and that, quite honestly, is something to be thankful for. So take these hacks and run with them like they're pilfered chips and you're a saucy seagull.

★ Ask a stranger what they're reading
★ Admit you're being a douche canoe
★ Look at the stars with your feet on the ground
★ Go on a social media diet
★ Write your work wife a thank-you note
★ Order a pizza
★ Change your heart rate
★ Watch an episode of *Toddlers & Tiaras*

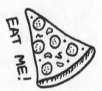

HOW TO LEVEL-UP FOR THE REST OF YOUR LIFE

Once you discover resilience, the really hard part is holding on to it. Because it's like a frog covered in coconut oil: it will do a stellar job of wriggling out of your grasp. Here's how to make that resilience stay put, forever.

CHAPTER TWENTY

Just like cave bae

(Or: Solve for happiness)

I want you to imagine you have an ice cube. A big, fat, juicy one. One that takes both hands to hold. Most people around you don't have any ice, so they're a little bit in awe of your frosty block. You're pretty happy with it yourself. It gives you pleasure and status and keeps you cool when things get a little hot under the collar.

But, as ice tends to do, eventually it melts. You don't notice it at first – you're too busy enjoying the easy chill your block affords you. But soon all you're left with is a puddle at your feet.

The problem is, now you know exactly what having an ice cube is like. It's more glorious than sex with an oiled-up demigod and you want it again.

So what do you do? You try to find another block of ice. You search in nooks and crevices and crannies, behind suitcases and under small animals. Before you know it, you're spending your ice-less days just dreaming about that time you had a cube of your own. Occasionally, you scroll through Instagram and see other people with their ice cubes – grinning widely, like they're mocking you. Your mind is occupied with the thought of how you could be crazy enough to let the one block you had melt in the first place. What you wouldn't give for just ONE MORE DAY WITH YOUR ICE CUBE!

Sounds a little intense, right … it's just ice? But this is basically how happiness works. You have it, you lose it, you mourn it, you want it again, it eludes you, you become obsessed with it. But happiness is a lot more like ice than you think – impermanent by its very nature. It's not meant to be forever – it's fleeting out in the real world, and trying to make it everlasting only ruins the time you have with it in the first place. It is an absurd, chase-our-tails scenario.

My advice to the ice-obsessed would be to try not to think about the cube itself, but what it's made from: hydrogen and oxygen. The elements that make up not only ice but water, steam, part of the air we breathe and the very atmosphere itself. It has so many iterations. You're quite literally surrounded by the components that make up your precious ice twenty-four hours a day – you just don't know how to appreciate it.

Happiness is exactly the same. Instead of focusing on that tangible, in-your-face chunk of happiness, pay more attention to its parts, the more abstract units you normally take for granted. The roof over your head, the sister who texts just to check in, the breakfast that started your day. These are all things you'd miss like limbs if you didn't have them. Just ask someone who doesn't and they'll tell you. The parts of your happiness are all around you if you just pay more attention.

So, in fact, it's not finding happiness that's the issue, or even holding on to it; it's simply knowing what it looks like. That's our real problem. We suck at it.

Because happiness, as we see it in the twenty-first century, is the solve to a problem. The problem is our lives. The solve, we figure, usually involves money. With money I could pay a personal trainer and get really skinny. Being skinny would mean more people would be attracted to me. Being attractive will lead to love. Love will make me happy. Being rich will ergo make me happy. It's bonkers, expecting your happiness to come from a barter system we invented. It's like expecting Bitcoin to help you fall pregnant or diamonds to cure your cancer. Money is helpful, of course – necessary even. But it's not a foolproof path to happiness.

So happiness, partially at least, is being at peace with the fact you'll never truly be completely happy. Not in the way you imagine. Not in the end of *Star Wars: Episode VI* kind of way.

The absolute biggest joy of having cancer (yes, I did say 'joy') was that I had a single predicament. I went from worrying about paying the bills; fretting about my career; driving myself bonkers about superannuation contributions; chasing love, a tighter behind and a million other entanglements to just one issue – surviving. That was all I had to do. I didn't have to worry about renewing my car insurance or watching my cholesterol – I didn't even have to worry about my taxes. My accountant blissfully put everything on hold for me until I finished treatment. No taxes for the malignant! The silver linings of cancer treatment aren't many, but that was one of them. Every possible burden I could have agonised about was now Future Emma's problem. Unless I didn't make it – then I'd never have to worry about them at all. What luck! No, all I had to do was get through it. And that brought with it a clarity like I've never experienced before. Everything extraneous was gone in an instant, as if washed away by some invisible sun shower. It was a *Walden*-esque epiphany. Only I still had running water and microwave popcorn.

When all you have to do is survive – and then you do – you're given something of a do-over. A chance to change what life looks like for you. If you choose not to wallow in your adversity, you get a whole new springboard. And I'm far from the only one who's used survival as such a platform.

'One story that comes to my mind is of a young woman who was kidnapped by a Caribbean gang and forced into prostitution. She ended up crossing her pimp and was finally ordered to dig her own grave. After months of captivity – and watching a friend who was similarly ordered to dig her own grave be shot and killed – she managed to escape. This woman had been traumatised on so many levels and yet, with help, she has since completely rebuilt her life. She's haunted by her past at times, but she made a conscious decision to move beyond what many might consider too overwhelming to manage.'

That's Lisa Cypers Kamen recounting a particularly memorable tale from her time as something of a positive pathfinder and happiness expert, a job which comes as a result of her master's degree in spiritual psychology. Lisa hosts a podcast called *Harvesting Happiness Talk Radio*. Which I love even exists. She's also an author, speaker, TEDx Talk–giving type who specialises in finding happiness after trauma. She's also spent some time coaching soldiers returning from war zones – the most cut-and-dry survival situation we know.

'They might think of themselves as weak or broken when they return home from the battlefield, but, in my experience, soldiers are some of the most resilient, highly intuitive, mindful and spiritual people I've met. I've witnessed incredible transformations in servicemen and women when they're supported with the validation that what they saw or did in combat might have been horrible, but it needn't brand them forever.'

Cancer, kidnapping and combat are all very different kettles of salmon, of course. But when all you can do in a given setting is survive, you learn pretty quickly everything outside of that is a choice. Just as with happiness, it's not about avoiding the trauma as much as it is about treating it as something that's transitory.

'Trauma is a natural byproduct of exposure to extraordinary amounts of stress,' says Lisa. 'The post-traumatic stress response is our body and brain doing exactly what they were designed to do – attempting to protect ourselves when overloaded.'

Give in to any one emotion in its entirety and your survival will be threatened. Moving out of survival mode then means some very conscious and deliberate choices about how you want to live going forward. Some people decide to climb on top of the experience; others decide to crawl up inside it – but everyone is changed by it.

'Nothing is a guarantee except the constancy of change – attitude is everything and wherever we focus our attention is where we find ourselves,' agrees Lisa. 'The only difference between happy and unhappy people is not the amount of hardship they've experienced, it's the relationship with their adversity.'

For the record, Lisa has had some experience with anguish herself. Which you kind of want in your trauma coach, to be fair.

'I strive to lead by example,' she says. 'During the recession I went through a divorce, lost all my financial resources and even my job due to my employer dropping dead of a heart attack. I found myself alone and homeless with two kids and my life ahead of me. The universe challenged me to walk my happiness talk. I took what I knew and put it into action to transcend and transform a very difficult set of multiple circumstances that were not working in my favour and I *thrived because of them.*'

Some people use optimism in the face of adversity; others find it afterwards. But anyone going through trauma knows it has to come eventually, because it's the only way out of the torture chamber you find yourself in.

This might be something you're struggling with at this very moment. If it is, the light at the end of the tunnel is almost non-existent. It is, quite simply, excruciating. Lisa and I also see eye to eye on the best way to start the trek towards the shiny end, though – throw a great, big shindig.

Now try this: throw a pity party

'I encourage a big juicy pity party full of tears, drama and the full gamut of emotions,' Lisa says. 'Being able to "get it out", preferably in the presence of someone who will truly listen to us, can be very therapeutic because as humans we yearn to be seen, heard and understood. Having empathetic and compassionate validation that our predicament truly is hard by another human being actually helps start the healing process. So I say have a fine whine or two or three and then redirect that energy into a solution. Stewing in our own juices ultimately does not make us feel better and, in fact, can contribute to righteous indignation at the unfairness of our sorrows.'

A whine or two, or a wine or four. Who's counting? But I promised you actionable steps and I'm not kidding around. The promise of talking about your problems for hours on end might not be enough to entice a friend around on its own (shocking), so, if you're inclined, add cocktails. My personal go-to is the espresso martini – the perfect accompaniment for discussing your damage. I've done this a few times and my recipe goes like this:

- One and a half shots of vodka
- One shot of espresso
- Half a shot of coffee liqueur
- Half a shot of simple syrup
- Shake over ice and serve.

If you're feeling especially fancy, a grain or two of sea salt really takes it up a notch. Although if you're going to spend the afternoon crying into your glass, you probably won't need the extra salt.

It's also entirely possible you're not a drinker – maybe tea is more your style. Or hot chocolate. Or kombucha. It really doesn't matter what it is. Medical professionals would probably tell you it's not great to be drinking alcohol in a heightened emotional state anyway. I wholeheartedly agree – I just also live in the real world. We have vodka out here and sometimes it's better than duct tape for patching breaches quickly.

But the more exciting step is actually the next one. It's the one that will really turn the healing up to eleven. You just have to start small. Real small.

Once your pity party is over and you've scrubbed the sticky martini residue off your kitchen bench (trust me, it'll happen), decide what you're going to do for the next hour.

That's it. That's all you need to do. This is essentially all I did for a whole year during treatment. This hour: I will get out of bed. Next hour: shower. After that: episode of *Battlestar Galactica*. Tiny one-hour pockets of action you have to get through.

Don't think more than three or four pockets ahead. Our big human brains are extremely clever – they can play out a situation in eight directions simultaneously – and because we're so creative each scenario is often fictionalised to the point they're more Dali than Rembrandt. Fast forward too far and you'll find yourself paralysed by the thought of a terrifying future that probably won't happen. That could not be less useful to you right now.

'The first and most powerful tool is definitely structure and schedule,' agrees Lisa. 'Creating a daily program or road map to follow is essential to just help support movement through the day. This might well be an hour-by-hour pursuit early on in the recovery process. A 7 am rise and shine, meditation, morning hygiene, breakfast, exercise, emails, et cetera. Break the day down into achievable steps so you can feel good about accomplishing them.'

Several times, my pockets would read more like a pre-schooler's than an adult's. Nap, it would say. Snack. Go outside. Brush Gloria's hair. (Gloria was my wig, not my Barbie doll, but you see the similarities.) And it worked. Suddenly I'd gone from planning my own funeral to planning a trip to the local cafe. If that went well, maybe next week I'd consider finding a pocket for the pub.

And make sure to add people – integrate them into as many pockets as you can. Phone calls, coffees, professional chitchat – even just texts. I would dedicate several pockets a week to simply responding to people who had enquired after the state of my boobs. Like I imagine Christina Hendricks has to do on occasion.

In this way, training your brain requires little more than a set of super simple equations, much like losing weight. More energy in than out, we'll put on weight. More out than in, the reverse happens. Happiness is almost boringly similar. The more energy you put into the process, the more you get out. Just like replacing unhealthy eating habits, repeat several times daily until you get into the swing of it. Your hourly chunks are like carrot sticks for the soul.

'If we approach our challenges like a mathematical problem by identifying known elements and missing pieces, we can then develop a strategy for solving the equation,' says Lisa. 'I once heard this great quote by Alan Cohen: "Every minus is half of a plus, waiting for a stroke of vertical awareness." Because you see, it's not the problem that's the real problem, it's our relationship with the problem that's the problem! It's important to call a spade a spade. What I mean by that is truthfully acknowledging that what's happening is unpleasant, painful, frightening and sad – be willing to confront the discomfort, then get busy building a structure to support the process of repair.'

Of course, just like regular maths, this comes easier to some than to others. I might be slick at optimism, but I flunked general maths at university. Twice. The third time I passed with a solid forty nine per cent pass conceded. It mightn't seem particularly impressive, but, technically, it's a win. You just have to do the same thing with gratitude.

'It's challenging to make a pessimistic person suddenly optimistic, but we can unlearn old behaviours and replace them with more optimistic ones through repetitive practice. This is where many people fail – they're simply unwilling to practise. There's also a theory the brain has a predisposed negativity bias that's a holdover from the caveman era. Early humans were hypervigilant because they were in fear of being eaten by a sabre-toothed tiger all the time. We're not being chased by animals, but our bodies respond in that same fight-or-flight mode. That mode includes negativity because it helps keep us on alert.'

Just like cave bae, we can't be lackadaisical when it comes to fending off foe.

'There's no room for physical or emotional laziness if we want change,' says Lisa.

Same-same but different.

'We have to practise the attributes of happy people. Gratitude, connected social relationships, having a sense of purpose, good self-care and spiritual practice, whatever that means to you, whether that's praying or gardening. All that gives a sense of being a part of something greater than one's self, and probably the most important power tool we own – controlling our attitudes.'

It sounds hard and convoluted because it is. But think about picking up a violin and trying to teach yourself to play from scratch. It's not going to be pretty. At least not until you've had a hell of a lot of practice and more than a few butt-clenchingly bad false starts. Surely having someone to copy would make that process a lot easier?

Same goes for this. Think: what would Dory do? Okay, referencing an animated fish is probably only going to get you so far. But find yourself a happiness role model. Because faking it till you make it works just as well with happiness as it does with resumés.

The lines in the sand are far blurrier than they are with learning an instrument, though. With the violin, you have tests and grades and recitals. With happiness, at best you have someone saying, 'You seem like you're doing really well lately.'

How will you know when you've really, truly graduated? When you can look at your trauma and honestly say you don't want to give it back. That's real end-of-the-movie, credits-rolling stuff.

'Personally, I've never met a person who has successfully triumphed over their demons, myself included, who say they'd trade their story for someone else's – because they learned X, Y and Z about themselves and it gave birth to their purpose as a result,' says Lisa. 'We need to learn to embrace that if we're alive, we'll have adversity. No one gets out of this life without it. But if we show up for life open, curious, heartfelt and focused, we're better equipped to handle what comes our way. Most people would say they didn't invite trauma into their lives, but when they conquered it, they became self-actualised and therefore have some nod of gratitude to that difficult situation for birthing their best self.'

Anyone else just picture themselves giving birth to themselves? If you didn't, you are now. Isn't that one for the Freudians? But she's right – once you can swim through the soup of your trauma and look back at it from the rim of the bowl, it will actually feel a lot like a rebirth. In the most cinematic sense of the word.

'Each of us will eventually have the opportunity to become the hero of our own lives because the hero story is only activated when he or she accepts the call to adventure. This call requires we be willing to undergo a metaphoric death – the giving up of some old aspect of ourselves – in order to be reborn. And it's only because of those challenges that the hero rises.'

See, now you're a hero. It just gets better and better. In the end, happiness is not the problem. Your situation isn't even the problem. The problem is you think they should be easier than they are. But it will get a lot less painful in a very short space of time with daily practice, an hour at a time. As Lisa would say, it should leave you 'pregnant with optimism about the possibilities ahead'. That's definitely coach speak for 'bloated on the fries at the bottom of the bag of life'. A contentment that may only be temporary, but damned if it isn't delicious while it lasts.

For something even more durable, you'd have to actually change how your genes are expressed. Possible? You betcha.

CHAPTER TWENTY-ONE

Winner winner, chicken dinner

(Or: Health and kindness)

Almost every religion that's ever held a gathering extolls the virtues of kindness to your fellow man. And, in a lot of instances, animals, plants and anything living. It almost seems like ground zero should you want to start a movement.

'Okay, guys, we've got the "Be nice to everyone" thing down ... what's next? Should we put in no sleeping around? Utah, I'm looking at you.'

The big five – Christianity, Judaism, Buddhism, Hinduism and Islam – have, despite their differences, a lot in common. The strongest thread being a sense of community. Why is this so important? Because humans need to belong. We crave it. We require it for our very survival. Kindness is important because it's what keeps communities humming. We've known it for thousands upon thousands of years. Fast forward to now, and we know it's paramount for personal health too. Get a load of this ...

A recent psychological experiment showed that doing acts of kindness for others leads to *actual changes in immune cell gene expression associated with disease resistance*. Literally: do something nice for someone else and feel better. This is almost tennessine-level brilliance if you ask me.

Just one more time for those who weren't paying attention: don't be a dick and you won't get sick.

As such, I suggest perhaps a lot of us have the pursuit of happiness all wrong. We spend so much time introspecting when the quickest way to get a hit is *by doing something for someone else*. Most of the time it doesn't even matter how big the thing is; sometimes the tiniest of actions is all it takes.

Hold the door open for someone: feel good.

Tell a stranger you like their boots: feel good.

Buy someone who needs it a meal: feel good.

Focusing on yourself is ultimately not where it's at. At least in terms of a more constant state of contentment. You will never be happy all of the time and you will most definitely never be perfect. What you can be, however, is kind. Your brain pays dividends on kind. It's so effective for making you feel good, it's like knowing which horse is going to win ahead of time; an almost guaranteed winner winner, chicken dinner.

But what happens when holding car doors open and paying for someone's coffee become a drop in the ocean? Because kindness – like anything else that makes you feel good – can be addictive. And suddenly what helped keep you buoyant before doesn't work any more. You need something stronger.

This is where altruism comes in. That would be larger-than-anyone-person, world-changing kindness. The variety you commit to for life as a self-actualised person. Which brings me very swiftly to my favourite asteroid nut. This mightn't seem the chapter for space science, but trust me, it is. Because Michael Dello-Iacovo – PhD candidate, lover of science-fiction and rock aficionado – is actually a lot like you. Other than the fact he spends his professional time figuring out how we might deflect an asteroid headed for Earth should we need to. Which could well happen.

'Yeah – any day, unfortunately.'

We have near misses all the time, apparently. We just don't always hear about them.

'Yesterday, we actually had a meteor come really close.'

Comforting.

But when he isn't spending his time gazing at space bodies, Michael is an effective altruist – and he thinks you should be too.

'Altruism means a few different things to people, but I think everyone would broadly agree it's the idea of wanting to have a positive impact with our life with the limited time and resources we have. To be an *effective* altruist, it makes sense to try and think carefully about what we do with that time and those resources in order to have as much positive impact as we can.'

When most people think of altruism, they tend to think about donating to charity. And it does include charity, of course – there are several organisations that do the hard work for you by rating the effectiveness of various charities online (givewell.org is a great example). But like anything else in modern life, it's not as easy peasy lemon squeezy as it is hard hard citrus yards. And according to Michael, charity isn't even the half of it.

'It could also mean asking yourself, "What kind of career should I take? What sort of job do I think would be impactful? What should I do with my spare time?" So just the idea that it's combining charity and rationality, the heart and the mind.'

As both the former CEO of Effective Altruism Australia and the host of a podcast called *Morality is Hard*, Michael is under no illusion these ideas are simple for people to adhere to. But when I say he's just like you, he is. He's not a millionaire or a business owner or a celebrity or even necessarily particularly decisive. He's just a guy trying to get through life by earning a living and doing his bit along the way. The only difference is, he's far more dedicated to doing his bit than the rest of us.

'For example, I've pledged to give everything I make over $45,000 each year for life to the world's most effective charities and causes.'

Are the producers of *The Bachelor* looking for a new candidate? I think I found him. Who would have thought a space scientist would be an overachiever? But it's not a number Michael just came to overnight.

'I saw friends I met through the effective altruism community making pledges like donating five per cent of their income per year, things like that. And I thought, yep – that's great, I'm going to get on to that. At the time I was living what I thought was a great life. I had a very high quality of living, but I was still only spending around $25,000 a year. So eventually I thought, wow – there's this huge gap between what I'm spending and need to be saving, and what I'm actually earning. And I realised I could be doing something really good with that.

'The reason I made the pledge public has a lot to do with an individual named Robert Wiblin who does a lot of blogging and writing about this online. He said that to give, to make a donation, or to perform an altruistic act and tell everyone about it is generally considered a selfish thing to do. But he thinks the selfish thing would be to tell no one about it. Because while we live in a society where people don't want to publicise acts of altruism, if you talk about it you actually encourage altruism in other people; you perpetuate giving norms.'

Almost-Doctor Mike has a point. And probably some incredibly robust immune cell gene expressions. But what about when money is tighter than a sixteenth-century mother superior? As it is for a hefty chunk of people around the world.

'I think charity is the one form of altruism that gets the most publicity and people think about the most,' says Michael. 'But you can also think about how to improve the world in other ways – I've even taken that as far as my diet. I adopted a vegan lifestyle in order to positively influence the environment and the lives of animals.'

I think maybe Disney should base their next prince on Michael, he's almost too good to be true.

But perhaps veganism isn't for you – maybe you need me to go even smaller still? I can do that. What about just not holding grudges? That won't cost you a cent *and* you can still have scrambled eggs for breakfast.

'I happen to think big picture, but altruism can be very small picture as well. And not holding grudges is actually something I feel really strongly about,' says Michael. 'When I was younger I'd hold grudges, but eventually I came to this realisation [that] we're all a product of so many different things – of genetics and upbringing for starters, and those two things we can't change. This became really obvious to me when I started to talk publicly about veganism and animal advocacy and certain people had very negative reactions to it. I realised they weren't necessarily choosing to get upset – they're just the product of so many different things, only part of which is their own decision. If someone does something to slight me now, in the moment it's easy to think about being combative – but I just remind myself to show them as much kindness as I can.'

So, Disney honchos, I'm thinking the prince should be called Apollo and wear tiny gold-plated asteroids as buttons.

I, on the other hand, am neither giving thousands of dollars a year nor ixnaying lamb chops. I did find my way to altruism through cancer, though, which a lot of people do. And thanks to a wrenching bombshell I'll get to later, I've given more in the months since I was diagnosed than every day before it combined. During treatment I had far less money than usual, mind you – even in a country with socialist healthcare, going through cancer isn't exactly financially beneficial. But I gave more time than I knew was possible – to fundraising endeavours, to teaching, to listening, to strangers. The idea of a more cavernous kindness suddenly worked for me because I was donating that time to something I cared a whole lot about. Which might seem almost self-serving – obviously the breast cancer patient wants to help find a cure for breast cancer. But it stuck. In a way that no other form of big-picture altruism had stuck with me before. The noise of all those charity phone calls and street canvassers died down and instead of avoiding it all like social ebola, I actually picked something and ran with it. But there's a reason nothing might have piqued your particular interest thus far.

'There's this idea of analysis paralysis where there are so many different factors influencing your decisions you feel like you can't really make a decision at all,' says Michael. 'We have to recognise there's a lot of uncertainty in what we do and just try to make the best decisions we can.'

So what does that look like when you haven't contracted a hideous disease or had someone die under avoidable circumstances? Michael suggests just figuring out what you spend a lot of time thinking about. Maybe you start every morning with a swim at the beach and therefore have a vested interest in marine conservation. Maybe you're a teacher who sees far too many children falling behind and wants to do their bit for literacy health. There's always something knocking around in your noggin.

'Then maybe try something small, like giving one per cent of your income to a charity over the course of a year and just see how you feel about that. From there you can work up to something like Giving What We Can, an effective altruism organisation that encourages people to pledge ten per cent of their income to support a charity financially over the course of their life. Or it might not be financial – it might be I want to spend ten hours volunteering this year.

'Whatever it is, rather than just thinking, "I want to be a good person," pick a specific goal. Find one concrete example of what you're going to do. And then at the end of the year you can go back and review, "Have I done that?" Maybe you have and you found it was actually very easy and you enjoyed it and then you can do a little bit more next year.

'I'm a very big fan of setting altruistic goals, particularly annual goals. I try and review mine every year and look back and see how I did according to what I wanted to do at the start of the year and whether there were any reasons I didn't quite make that. Just be very clear with yourself this is the one thing you're going to do this year to try and improve the lives of others.'

You've heard all this in some form or another before, of course – give more, want for less. But your resources for altruism are far more plentiful than you probably imagine.

'Resources can be time, money, energy, your network, your friends and family.'

Maybe you know a guy who knows a guy who can print pamphlets really cheap.

'Sometimes giving something like that to help a local event get off the ground, while a much smaller application, could actually be more impactful.

'You have to think in terms of long-term sustainability. It makes no sense to be altruistic to the point of sacrifice – being super altruistic for three years and burning out is nowhere as good as being consistently altruistic in the long-term. And if you start to feel regret, I think you need to look at if you're doing too much. But for me, helping other people brings me a lot of happiness. And it's a monetary sacrifice, but I think the sacrifice versus what I get from it makes it all well and truly worth it. I can't imagine going back – altruism is just something I do now without thinking about it.'

Michael's top tip? Find a tribe that subscribes to something with pride.

'I think there's something to be said for the sort of people you surround yourself with. You tend to become more like them. So if you have this idea of the sort of person you want to be, surround yourself with similar minds. Not so similar that you're not challenged, but people you can learn from. Finding a mentor can also be really good. When I first started getting involved in altruism, I found someone who taught me everything she knew and I will be forever grateful to her. I wouldn't be the person I am today without that education.'

Okay, at this point you might be wondering what all this has to do with your trauma. Once you've dealt with the more pressing pieces of the puzzle that is your adversity, however, this represents one of the final rungs on the ladder of resilience. Because you won't ever realise how small your life is – and therefore your problems are – until you take a step back and help other people in need. As soon as you do that, everything – ironically – feels bigger. And an affinity for other people is key to your ability to snap back next time something upsets your status quo. Because people matter more than money. People matter more than being right. *People matter more.* I don't know how to say that with any more emphasis.

Now try this: **take your mum to bingo**

Ask anyone who's dying – read letters on the internet penned by terminally ill patients if you don't happen to have a chronically diseased pal lying around – and you'll see the common thread. The thing they're thankful for, and wish they had spent more time on, is always people. Kindness to other people should be your legacy far before trust funds and watches. Even if you just dedicate yourself to taking your dad to the movies, popping in on an elderly neighbour or driving your mum and her friends to bingo once a week for those sweet disease-resistant gene expressions, just do *something*.

'There's a lot to be said for small acts and big acts feeding off each other. If you're living altruistically in your everyday, doing these small actions just comes naturally, and vice versa. You start asking yourself, "How can I help as many people as possible?" Just make sure you're thinking about the impact. I know some people just think about how much money is going into a project – a lot of people and organisations just rate charities purely on their overhead cost – but that's not actually always the best way to judge effectiveness.'

This is actually something you'll come across when you get involved with charity – the varying ideas of a board or an organisation won't always gel with yours. And some people get frustrated to the point of quitting altogether. Stick it out. Be better than that. Be selfish about it if you have to. Remind yourself you're there for your own self-actualisation, your own boosted immune cells, your own emotional growth. Which, in that lottery syndicate kind of way, is actually a win for all because you're helping other people in the process.

As a religious and even spiritual decree, kindness is unfortunately something we've diluted. We're kind, all right ... as long as it's to people who look like us, think like us and talk like us. So perhaps, through our collective trauma, we can take this opportunity to update the mindset. Kindness doesn't have to be about soup kitchens or monthly donations – it can be as simple as working with or reaching out to someone who's different from you and seeing what you can add to each other's lives. This is something a lot of people actively avoid doing on a daily basis. We are all far more xenophobic than we'd generally like to admit.

But trauma is the great leveller. It does not discriminate, not for anyone. Cancer doesn't care what colour you are; your miscarriage didn't happen because you're Jewish; and your mum didn't die as a result of you wearing a hijab. Trauma can come for you any time with or without your consent. Having people be kind to you during this period will obviously make the impact far easier to bear. And that's the other side of the kindness coin – not just the giving but the receiving. It's easy to think of altruism as something you do for others, but you have to let other people in with the same fervour.

Which brings me to how altruism found me.

It was the day I found out I needed chemo and lots of it. A rough day. Up until this point, still the worst day of my life. Quite frankly I hope it never gets knocked off its perch.

My mother and one of my best friends had both come with me to the appointment that morning, and understandably neither of them really knew what to say. 'That sucks' and 'We'll get through it' didn't really compute. When we got to my apartment, I told them I wanted to be alone, and shut my bedroom door behind them.

As I lay in bed at 2 o'clock in the afternoon, tears pooling in my ears, I tried desperately to assimilate this new information. I'm just going to keep this to myself, was my conclusion. Having the world know about it will make it far grander and more public than it needs to be. I'll tell my family, of course, and a handful of friends, but if I just get a great melon rug once my hair falls out, no one will be any the wiser.

This is something a lot of people who find their health threatened tend to do. When even your own body isn't under your control any more, your first instinct is to hold on to the last thing you *can* control: the dissemination of information. Being the authority on who finds out and when, and how much they know, is something you want to seize with both hands like a Madonna clutching her child.

After I had made that decision, I just cried myself to sleep. Something I hadn't done since I was twelve years old and my mother sent me to bed without dinner. A punishment I received for refusing to eat what she had made for dinner, ironically.

An hour later, I was awoken from the type of heavy-slumber you can really only achieve by sobbing until you pass out. I'd forgotten to set my phone to silent and it was yapping at me like an electronic puppy that wanted to go outside. I went to turn it off, but even a quick glance was enough to tell me something was askew. I had tens of messages. Dozens. And they were still coming in. 'I just heard about the chemo, I'm so sorry.' This from a friend I hadn't seen since her wedding a year earlier. 'OMG, I just read about it on Facebook. I can't believe this is happening. Sad face emoji!' From another I'd last greeted almost a decade ago.

What the actual, mother-loving fuck. My confusion at the situation I'd just been thrust into was so bulky I had trouble knowing where to look, what to do with my hands.

I sat upright on the end of the bed and texted my friend – the one who had come with me to the appointment. *Did you put something on Facebook?* Not me, she said, I would never. *Did you email anyone?* Nope, didn't email anyone. Curiouser and curiouser.

'Oh, wait …' she said. And then she told me that one of our other friends called to see how it went. 'And I told her – could that be it?'

Yes. Yes, I think it could.

It only took three more text messages for the whole story to unfold. When this friend had heard about my chemo, she was upset. Devastated, actually – that someone she loved was going to have to go through something so harrowing. And her first instinct was to help. In any way she could. So – it being the age for kickstarters of all kinds – she started a crowdfunding page. One designed to pay for the wig I'd need now that I was going to be balder than a freshly laid egg. She shared it with ten people who shared it with another ten people … and an hour later, hundreds of eyes had drunk it in.

I was fuming. I found myself so angry at her, at everyone, that I was shaking. The salt grain–sized smidge of control I thought I had left had been ripped away from me while I was sleeping.

It took me a few days to be able to talk to her again. More still to get used to the fact people I hadn't spoken to in years felt the need to donate money to my plight. I already had cancer and didn't much want to feel like a charity case on top of that.

Which is around about the time I realised I was being A GIANT ASSHOLE CASSEROLE.

Not only was I not acting altruistically towards others, I wasn't even accepting the altruism that was being directed towards me. What kind of asshattery is that? So after letting the ninety-eight people who were benevolent enough to care to buy me a wig – which was utterly glorious by the way, and made from my own hair, which I largely harvested before it fell out – I set to work on no longer being such a ball wrinkle in the lap of life. I helped more, complained less. I stopped being too proud to accept help and too busy to offer it. I became an effective altruist before I even knew what the term meant. And all because someone cared enough to be frantically kind in my direction.

It's easy to think you won't ever need that kind of charity, and sometimes accepting it can be harder than giving it, but it's all part of the same ball of ethical wool. And whichever side of the yarn you find yourself on, you will be happier if you embrace the messiness of compassion.

'I absolutely consider it a moral obligation, but I also get a lot of happiness from it as well,' agrees Michael. 'It's the perfect coincidence. Everyone I know who does this is happier after making it a core part of their life.'

If not for me, do it for Prince Apollo.

Or yourself, really. That's probably the best option.

If happiness is something you want in your life with more regularity than your current bowel movements, you're going to need to do this. Once you do, you're ready for the final level of the working-through-your-trauma tower. It's worth it, I promise – there's even seafood involved.

CHAPTER TWENTY-TWO

14 inches,
or 35.56 centimetres

(Or: Maximise your
emotional intelligence)

I recently had a fallout with my web browser. Had she – I don't know why my browser is a she, she just is – had she been a real person, we would've undoubtedly exchanged strongly worded text messages before ignoring each other for several days, only to come to the conclusion we had no one else to watch re-runs of *Frasier* with, at which point we would've sheepishly forgiven each other and moved on.

Only she isn't a real person, so it was far more frustrating.

She'd developed this baffling habit of refreshing my inbox while I was in the middle of reading things, sending emails before I'd finished writing them and generally being a real Jeff Goldblum–sized fly in my ointment. When a for-real friend pointed out that maybe it was because I was running my emails in a browser window, I looked at him quizzically. And when I say 'friend', I mean My Great Experiment. That's right, he went the distance –

through chemo and beyond. So I decided to keep him. Well, it was probably more a mutual decision, really, but it's all in how you frame it.

'I'm just saying that you wouldn't have those problems if you just used the mail application on your computer,' he said, like he was teaching his great-grandmother how to play Microsoft Solitaire.

Was he right? Surely it was a Mary-Kate v Ashley situation. Six of one, half a dozen of the other. Although now that he'd pointed it out, doubt was creeping in. Why had I never considered using the application *built specifically for this task* before?

'I guess ... well, I guess I've just always done it this way,' I replied.

And that little edict right there might actually be the most dangerous sentence in the English language.

If you had to be really honest about why you haven't changed cities or jobs or partners, even though deep down you have an inkling you're destined for a different one, wouldn't the answer likely be: because this is what I'm used to? It's easy, it's comfortable. *I've just always done it this way.*

This is one of those key things mentally strong people just don't do with any real frequency. In the scientific tradition of excluding people by using acronyms for almost everything, psychologists often refer to this as high EI or EQ. That would be emotional intelligence or emotional quotient. It essentially describes the ability of a person to recognise not only their own emotions but those of others. To label those emotions and then react to them appropriately. To let emotions guide their decisions and behaviour, and be aware of how those same emotions affect other people's decisions and behaviour. Those with a high EQ are the anti-psychopaths of the world. They're empathic, generally have increased mental health, often hold leadership roles and perform well in most areas in life.

Like every psychological hypothesis in the world, it has its pooh-poohers. But I'd say EQ is a better measure of a person than IQ. Of course, I'm not looking to fill the chair of Lucasian Professor at Cambridge,[2] so when it comes to scientific hypotheses of any kind, I'm really just going with my gut.

For example, a person with high emotional intelligence would realise they were letting their attachment to a chronic routine hinder them from a far more efficient modus operandi and change their actions accordingly. They'd use the flipping mail application, basically.

Times of great upheaval tend to shake these kinds of silly attachments loose, though, whether you like it or not. A breakup or a divorce in particular is often a cascade of these types of upheavals. First, you lose that person's presence. Then you lose their family. Their friends. The joint bank account. The half-dozen texts you got from them a day. A scapegoat for getting out of boring social situations. A place to spend Christmas. It's like a giant game of dominoes in which the tiles are all the pieces of your life, falling one after the other in a torrent that feels relentless. You're gaining things as well, of course, but those things are much harder to see when grief is all up in your grill.

As these things go by the wayside, however, all manner of tiny bad habits you took for granted fall away as well. The monotonous way you'd order the same Thai food every Friday night. Your laziness in never checking the mailbox. The fact you go to the same holiday house every Easter. Things you'd just always done. Things you're now realising don't have to be done that exact same way every time. As horrendous as it is, a process like this helps you tap back into your emotional intelligence – to pay attention to your feelings and use them to your advantage.

---

2   A role held by both Isaac Newton and Stephen Hawking, should that ever come up at trivia night.

My great upheaval was like a highlighter for all the things I'd always done while wishing for more – something we all know to be the first sign of stupidity. I did my hair the same way for a decade, for example. I also lived in the same apartment, did the same job, went on the same kind of holiday and, yes, even ate the same Thai food. My EI was telling me something was lacking, but it wasn't making me get off my rear end and change it.

Cancer, however, upended all of those things – every single one – in one wide brushstroke. And for that, I'm genuinely thankful for its savagery. Because I now pay a lot more attention to what my emotions are telling me before I act. They're like toddlers, remember – they crave attention. Give it to them and they'll thrive. Just make sure it's the good kind of attention, not the bad kind. Toddlers don't know the difference; they just want to be seen and heard. They'll smash your favourite mug for the attention if you let them.

'There's a notion out there that emotional intelligence is a soft skill or the tendency to be nice to people, but it's really something that enables you to make informed choices about how to manage yourself,' said Jacqueline Hinds when I probed her for the DL on EI.

She would know – she's a certified emotional intelligence coach, the chair of the Society of Emotional Intelligence in the UK, and board chair and international liaison for the International Society of Emotional Intelligence USA. And despite apparently holding more chairs than an IKEA catalogue, she's also very down to earth. Must be all that EI, TBH.

My favourite Jacqueline thought nugget just so happens to be about bullying.

'Bullying is a form of flattery,' she says. 'A back-handed compliment, yeah – but when people see things they don't possess, it irritates them. Rather than embrace it or learn from it, they let it get to them. What they then do is something to upset the person, to knock the shine off them. People who lack emotional intelligence, when they're in a situation where they're upset and they're projecting, what they tend to do is go into the corners and sweep up any little dust bunnies they can find, then pile them up to make something more substantive. When you start deconstructing it, it's like – oh my goodness, there's actually nothing here. Why are you so angry?'

Remember that before you get into an internet debate with a jerk who left something nasty lying under your latest Instagram photo. They're flattering you with dust bunnies. And this is exactly the kind of mental resilience we want to cultivate – the kind where you can turn the despotic actions of others into absurdities rather than letting them hammer at your self-esteem. Where trauma of all kinds just reflects off you like sunshine bouncing off well-oiled abs. Something an emotionally unintelligent person would probably bully you for having if you happened to possess them in the first place.

'When you're EI savvy, you'll find it a lot easier to engage with individuals,' says Jacqueline. 'I find it easier to help people work through and compartmentalise their issues or concerns, and get them to see the bigger picture in their present circumstance. Higher levels of emotional intelligence can also aid individuals going through mental crises such as depression and anxiety. This doesn't replace the much-needed mental-health advice and therapy that qualified professionals provide, but I do feel individuals with lower-level mental-health issues could benefit from learning how to tap into and build their confidence and competence around these skills.'

Well, show me a human being with perfect mental health and I'll show you a delusional pinhead. By which I mean – we all of us have something to learn in this arena. So I'm going to default to Jacqueline for this particular lesson because it's important, she really knows what she's talking about and I'm basically just an enthusiastic cretin with a keyboard.

In order to really tap into one's emotional intelligence, understanding the four basic components of EI is essential.

a) Self-awareness

This is considered the foundation for all the other components of emotional intelligence. Self-awareness means being conscious of the emotions within yourself at any given time.

b) Self-management

The second component of emotional intelligence is managing your emotions. Operationally it means an individual needs to be able to balance their own moods internally so that worry, anxiety, fear or anger don't ever get in the way of what needs to be done. Managing emotions doesn't mean suppressing or denying them, but understanding them and using that to deal with situations productively. Those who can manage their emotions perform better because they're able to think clearly.

c) Social awareness

Being socially aware simply means you understand how to react to different social situations and can effectively modify your interactions with other people to achieve the best results. It also means being aware of the world around you and how different environments influence different people. Increasing social awareness means improving the skills you use to connect with others verbally, nonverbally and in the community.

d) Relationship management

The final component of emotional intelligence is the ability to connect with others, build positive relationships, respond to their emotions and influence those around you. It's also vital in negotiating successfully, resolving conflicts and working with others toward a shared goal.

Okay, good speed schooling. Basically, you need to know when you're feeling like shit, be able to stop yourself from taking it out on other people, still be charming when the occasion calls for it and continue to get your job done.

'I'd also say emotionally intelligent people tend to have a way of bouncing back from challenges and forging ahead to pursue their goals despite adverse situations they may face,' says Jacqueline. So, that would be: exactly who we all want to be after reading this book.

But how do you practise emotional intelligence? It's not like just memorising lines in a textbook. Identifying emotions seems easy enough, right? I'm sad. I'm anxious. I'm hangry. But, of course, it's not quite that simple. And while we're at it, can you tell how your friend is feeling? Is he sad or depressed or listless or distracted or mad or just tired? And is that emotion incidental or integral to the situation? It's a hot mess, is what it is.

The answer to being more emotionally intelligent is simply pressing pause.

For instance, imagine you were counting a huge pile of beans. When you rush the job, it's easy to lose count. Then you have to start again. Then you get frustrated. Which makes you lose count again. Had you just stopped every now and again to write the number down, you could have divided the job into much more manageable chunks.

Emotional intelligence works in the same way. You simply have to teach yourself to pause and assess where you're at before going any further.

Now might be a good time to bust out that seafood.

'When you stop and work out what's triggering your emotions, you can teach yourself to assess the situation better,' says Jacqueline. 'It's a bit like being in a giant goldfish bowl – you're in there swimming around and every so often you need to do a spot check. So you stop and take a look around just to make sure you're still swimming around other goldfish, because sometimes these other emotions can creep in like so many little sharks and barracudas and piranhas. If you're not keeping track, you can get hijacked by them, eaten alive, without even knowing they're there. By the time you realise, it's too late.'

So if you don't want to be fish sticks, pay attention.

'If you take that moment to pause and look around, you can temper any situation. You can understand it and therefore tame it to the point you're not provoked. Then people can poke the bear, stroke him, jump on his back – none of it will worry you. You can almost predict the future because you get to the point you can actually see something before it happens, and you can stop yourself from losing it in the moment. I suppose in a sense it's like seeing a pothole. You know if you continue on that path you're going to fall in it. But if you go slightly to the left or to the right, you're going to able to avoid it.'

Now try this: recite the alphabet

Taking a moment was something I learned to do because I needed it to survive. When every other day someone is handing you bad news punctuated by phrases like 'survival rate' and 'infertility' and

'Your credit card's been declined again, ma'am', you simply can't give in to all the emotion that comes with it. You'd be a puddle. So you learn to pause and figure out what to do about each thing before you let any more information in. Which isn't easy. Not least of which because there's actually more than one reaction going on inside you in any given moment.

So when you find yourself in the eye of the storm, what do you do?

I would recite the alphabet to myself. Something that would take approximately fifteen seconds, which is a pause in and of itself. But I found it also short-circuited my stress response for a brief period, giving me enough time to breathe and assess a situation logically. An unsurprisingly useful skill in all areas of life.

'The heart and the brain are only separated by fourteen inches, but the conflict between them is the biggest battle going on inside anyone,' says Jacqueline. 'Think about something as simple as going shopping and saying to yourself, "I love those shoes." You can't help but want them, right?

'But then your head butts in and says, "Yeah, but you've got no money in the bank to pay for them."

'To which your heart replies, "Sure, but they'd look really nice on me and I could wear them to that party."

'And your head responds with, "But you've got no money in the bank."

'Then your heart says, "Yeah, but I can use my overdraft."

'Then your head replies, "Yeah, but then you've got to pay it back."

'It's just constant; they're always in conflict. Even over the smallest of things.'

She's right – these two giant organs are arguing with each other all day long. At best, you're just a giant meaty puppet for their discourse. Which is the real reason emotional trauma is so difficult to process. So much of it is unseen, it has no physicality. Your heart feels it all at once and your head is just shrugging its shoulders at the enormity of it all.

But nail emotional intelligence and those conversations sync up. They become more of a rational monologue than a cacophonous dialogue. And you'll know when you get there because other people will notice it. They won't know what they're noticing exactly, but I guarantee they'll point it out.

'When I think about it, people saw the difference in me before I saw it in myself,' said Jacqueline. 'They'd say, "Oh, you're really different." Oh, really? Because my hair is longer, my makeup is different? No, it was something else, but they didn't know what it was. It was only later I realised it was because my whole mindset had changed. I just don't get angry about stuff any more, I really don't. The Jackie of days gone by had a bit of a temper, was maybe even a bit of a scorpion. Now I've found the things that consistently impacted my time and attention, and heightened my frustration and stress levels, simply no longer take centre court.'

I had a similar experience. A friend of mine calls it 'The big chill'. Where I used to freak out and get upset and question the world and most of the men in it, I now just take everything at face value. It doesn't mean I don't find certain situations sub-optimal, but the fear doesn't touch me any more. I'm resilient and I know it. I can cheer myself up or calm myself down without needing an outside influence. And when you can do that for yourself, you'd be amazed at what you can do for other people.

'Once you actually get to that point, you can understand where someone's coming from, you can walk a mile in their shoes and you can take the sting out of any situation without ever raising your voice a decibel. Sometimes when you see a situation brewing, you know exactly what the end result is going to be, or what it's going to lead to, so you can channel certain things to make sure that if it does blow up, it's cushioned. You can get people to see the bigger picture. You can get them to understand the impact it's having on their head and their heart. Get them to see the turmoil, the fear, the anticipation – all the emotions bubbling up inside them.'

While cushioning emotional blows is a fairly choice skill to have, the most important thing emotionally intelligent people do is actually value *all* emotions. Positive, negative, and everything in between. They know anger is just as useful as elation, fear is just as powerful as love, and frustration is a call to action in the same way lust is. While I don't think anyone should wallow in an emotion that's making them question getting out of bed in the morning, all emotions serve a purpose. We idolise happiness for a reason, but it's not the only deputy in town. This is incredibly important to remember should you spend a lot of time around children, yours or otherwise. Scolding them for being sad or mad or grumpy isn't going to help them be happier, more positive beings. Getting them to understand why they feel that way and what actions they can take to feel differently is infinitely more helpful for them and far less profitable for their future shrink.

Our emotions aren't there to hinder us – quite the opposite; they give us an edge, a raison d'être; they are quite possibly the actual meaning of life. I don't mean to get all Monty Python on you, but an emotionless life would be so shallow I dare say it would be a valley of nihility.

But find your EI and you will find a calm you can take with you wherever you go for the rest of your days. And as a result, you'll be able to make more rational decisions to get you to where you want to go. You'll be able to avoid the potholes. You'll even be able to get your head and your heart to kiss and make up. This is one of humankind's most unique feats and it's there for the taking if you want it enough. You just have to stop doing things because that's how you've always done them. After that, everything else gets a whole lot easier.

CHAPTER TWENTY-THREE

A spoonful of sugar

(Or: How to unfuck yourself for good)

My final question is: how do you unfuck yourself for good?

It's certainly not an uncomplicated exploit. Once I wrapped up my cancer regimen, I started noticing all the meagre things I found so happy-inducing while I was sick – *the sun, the stars, the old lady that smiled at me in the lift!* – started losing their sheen. I worried that before too long, I would once again be stressing over bad hair days and parking fines. Paper cuts and the size of my thighs. I could feel some of my newfound exuberance slipping away and that was completely and utterly terrifying.

For many people, almost dying means finally catching on to what's worth living for – right at the eleventh hour when everything else slips away. When you get jerked back from the precipice, you have to hold on to that new-found knowledge, because it does a very good job of wanting to tiptoe back into oblivion. You find yourself hankering for that recent version of you – that humble, happy person you were for a brief time when you realised you were getting a second chance.

But near-death experience or not, we're all achingly aware any kind of enduring happiness is elusive. Trying to hold on to it for any length of time is like trying to keep sugar in a sieve. So sweet yet so capricious. But there are ways to keep it close; some simple, some more difficult. Some we've talked about in this book, several we haven't even touched on. But above all, we know we need water and light and shelter and friends to be at our best. We're essentially like really tall canines who walk on two legs and only sniff each other's genitals behind closed doors.

There is one device I find infinitely useful, though. One clever little way to keep the sugar this side of the sieve. This is the one that stopped my jubilance going the way of my eyebrows and I've saved it for last because it's so damn powerful.

Now try this: replace every 'I've got to' with 'I get to'

Instead of 'I've got to go to work ...', it's 'I get to go to work!' Instead of 'I've got to pick up the kids again today ...', it's 'I get to pick up the kids again today!' Instead of 'I've got to try to beat cancer today ...', it's 'I get to try to beat cancer today!' It's a midget-sized transition that yields Schwarzenegger-sized results. It's so simple yet so super-loaded with perspective. It wouldn't surprise me if one day we discover this little neurolinguistic trick lights up all the right parts of the brain in all the right places, the way a sky lights up on New Year's Eve. Using this little about-face will help create neural pathways that are grateful and generous and happy to be alive. It will make it very hard to complain about your lot in life and almost impossible to lament your cellulite. I use it every day in every way.

I managed to get to a place where I could happily wave goodbye to my imaginary parasitic twin and hello to my breast cancer tumour. It happened quickly because I forced it to. I chose to go through it instead of hanging on to the ledge like a damsel in distress waiting for a fictional hero with a magic solution. Should my cancer ever return, I hope I can do it all over again – this time with really buoyant breast implants and the knowledge I've done everything I possibly could.

It's the ultimate sure-thing that we're all going to meet our end sooner or later, and very few of us will get to choose when. Any illusion of control is just that. Quite literally, all you've got with any certainty is *right now*, so don't fritter it away maligning your yesterdays. That's such a monumentally wasteful activity. Being truly unfuckwithable means taking whatever inferno you find yourself in and walking right over the coals. You can't change it, you can only kick it in the balls until it screams at you to stop … at which time you obviously will because you're an enlightened person now.

But if you take one thing away from this book, make sure you do all of the above with the life vest that is other people. Because no one will be impressed that you did it alone – that you built that empire, walked that mountain, or beat that disease, alone. People have far more room in their rosy-coloured chest organ for people who need people. For people who bounce off and thrive on people. Be that person and stop pretending you can handle all your shit alone. I know strong people want to suffer in silence; I used to be one of them. If feels more wilful, more independent – less trouble for everyone else. But do that and you have no one to delight in your growth or watch you heal. All you will have is the knowledge you went it alone and that will die with you. Not even stoicism has an answer for that.

What you should be spending your time on is finding love. Not just romantic love, as alluring as it is. Having someone be the clip-on koala to your pencil is obviously a gratifying accomplishment, but what I mean is loving the pillow slip you sleep on. The sun that fades those sheets when you leave them out to dry. The patch of the world where that sun hits your face. The laughter that comes out of that face when you're with your friends. The friends that make all of that worthwhile. The world can be a terribly romantic place with or without someone to bump gonads with. So stop trying to do it all alone. Stop trying to do anything alone. This life was meant to be spent in the pursuit of others. Find the right people and even a coffee date will be an adventure fit for Dickens.

Know that finding those allies takes time. People aren't vending machines you can just put effort coins into until friendship drops out. But being kinder to everyone you come across – especially those who are different from you – will make it far more likely you'll stumble across your kin. And when it comes to being resilient to the curveballs that are hurtled in your direction, they will be the best weapons you have.

When I finished treatment and looked around, so much had changed. Almost everything, in fact. How I looked, where I lived, what I was doing with my life. There was an adjustment period. It was confusing. Almost discombobulating. Of course, I still have bad times, sad times and mad times. But they're just little bubbles which I know how to pop. And that usually means reaching out to someone I love – for help, for advice, for the sound of a human voice. Because the best thing about the worst days of your life is they show you who you want to spend the good ones with in glorious technicolour detail.

The bad news is what has happened to you has happened to you. The good news is it can stay in the past. None of what you have learned in this book is about trying to change who you are; it's not about making you more palatable or desirable to other people. It's important to know you are enough as you are right now without needing to change a thing. As soon as you realise that, the rest will be SO MUCH EASIER. Because it's only then you understand any growth is for you and you alone. For your happiness and contentment and not for the validation of anyone else.

Never feel flawed because you've experienced something traumatic. You are not a less covetable person because you've been through hell. A few small cracks along the way doesn't make you broken; it just makes you limited edition. So smile at yourself in the mirror, accept compliments gracefully, and stop trying to impress people you've never met with pictures of things you really should just be enjoying in real time.

If there's one final piece of advice I can give you, one last thing I learned from the Big C, it's this: don't ever, ever save anything – not the dinner plates, not the dress, not the cologne, not the apology, not the thank you, not the love letter and definitely not the good wine – for a special occasion.

Your life *is* your special occasion.

Live like it.

ACKNOWLEDGEMENTS

Funny-looking word, very important sentiment

Thank you to my father, Zoran Markezic, for tackling the beast before me so I knew what strength looked like. To my mother, Roslyn Markezic, for the insane levels of cooking, cleaning, changing of bandages and unconditional love. To my sisters, Claire Pawar and Jessica Snell, for the laughs, normality and champagne. And to my brothers-in-law, otherwise I'll never hear the end of it.

To Lucy Cousins for coming to every single appointment, dictaphone and notepad in hand, and never once saying 'Everything happens for a reason.' To Rebecca Whish for outing me with the fiercest affection I've ever known. To David Smiedt for his support of all kinds and especially for making me get up on stage. To Emma Vidgen, Matt Coyte, Alicia Pyke and Guy Mosel for the life-affirming dinner parties, my cousins for being some of the best that exist, Kerri Sackville for the Jewish penicillin, Angela Bishop for teaching me your story can always make a difference and Gemma Sutherland for making my boobs front-page news.

To Sanjay Warrier, Catriona McNeil, Ruth Mirto, Andy Hampson, Sarah Ferguson, Edith Maling, Shirley Baxter and the whole gang at the Chris O'Brien Lifehouse. I mean … #cancersquadgoals, seriously.

And, finally, to Kieran Ots – when everything was unabridged chaos, there you were. There's so much to thank you for I would hardly know where to start so I'm just going to pick one thing: thanks for having sex with me when I was horny, bald and had surgical tubes coming out of me. That was neat.